Exercise Testing in Pulmonary Hypertension and Heart Failure

Editor

SCOTT H. VISOVATTI

HEART FAILURE CLINICS

www.heartfailure.theclinics.com

Consulting Editor
EDUARDO BOSSONE

Founding Editor
JAGAT NARULA

January 2025 • Volume 21 • Number 1

ELSEVIER

1600 John F. Kennedy Boulevard • Suite 1800 • Philadelphia, Pennsylvania, 19103-2899

http://www.theclinics.com

HEART FAILURE CLINICS Volume 21, Number 1
January 2025 ISSN 1551-7136, ISBN-13: 978-0-443-13001-4

Editor: Joanna Gascoine
Developmental Editor: Nitesh Barthwal

Heart Failure Clinics (ISSN 1551-7136) is published quarterly by Elsevier Inc., 360 Park Avenue South, New York, NY 10010-1710. Months of publication are January, April, July, and October. Business and editorial offices: 1600 John F. Kennedy Boulevard, Suite 1800, Philadelphia, PA 19103-2899. Periodicals postage paid at New York, NY, and additional mailing offices. Subscription prices are USD 297.00 per year for US individuals, USD 100.00 per year for US students and residents, USD 324.00 per year for Canadian individuals, USD 341.00 per year for international individuals, and USD 100.00 per year for Canadian and foreign students/residents. For institutional access pricing please contact Customer Service via the contact information below. To receive student and resident rate, orders must be accompanied by name of affiliated institution, date of term, and the *signature* of program/residency coordinator on institution letterhead. Orders will be billed at individual rate until proof of status is received. Foreign air speed delivery is included in all *Clinics* subscription prices. All prices are subject to change without notice. Orders, claims, and journal inquiries: Please visit our Support Hub page https://service.elsevier.com for assistance.

Reprints. For copies of 100 or more of articles in this publication, please contact the Commercial Reprints Department, Elsevier Inc., 360 Park Avenue South, New York, NY 10010-1710. Tel.: 212-633-3874; Fax: 212-633-3820; E-mail: reprints@elsevier.com.

Heart Failure Clinics is covered in *MEDLINE/PubMed (Index Medicus)*.

Contributors

CONSULTING EDITOR

EDUARDO BOSSONE, MD, PhD, FCCP, FESC, FACC
Department of Public Health, Department of Internal Medicine, Interdepartmental Center for Gender Medicine Research (GENESIS), Cardiovascular Disease Fellowship Program, Cardiovascular Pathophysiology and Therapeutics (CardioPath) Ph.D Program, UNESCO Chair on Health Education and Sustainable Development, Faculty of Medicine - University of Naples "Federico II", Italy

EDITORS

SCOTT H. VISOVATTI, MD, FACC, FCCP
Director, Pulmonary Hypertension and Pulmonary Embolism Program, Clinical Associate Professor, Division of Cardiovascular Medicine, Department of Internal Medicine, The Ohio State University College of Medicine, Columbus, Ohio, USA

EDUARDO BOSSONE, MD, PhD, FCCP, FESC, FACC
Department of Public Health, Department of Internal Medicine, Interdepartmental Center for Gender Medicine Research (GENESIS), Cardiovascular Disease Fellowship Program, Cardiovascular Pathophysiology and Therapeutics (CardioPath) Ph.D Program, UNESCO Chair on Health Education and Sustainable Development, Faculty of Medicine - University of Naples "Federico II", Italy

AUTHORS

PRACHI P. AGARWAL, MD, MS
Clinical Professor, Radiology, Director, Cardiothoracic Radiology, Division of Cardiothoracic Radiology, Department of Radiology, University of Michigan, Ann Arbor, Michigan, USA

VIKAS AGGARWAL, MD, MPH
Senior Staff, Division of Cardiovascular Medicine, Department of Internal Medicine, Henry Ford Hospital, Detroit, Michigan, USA

CHRISTIAN BASILE, MD
Researcher, Division of Cardiology, Department of Medicine, Karolinska Institutet, Solna, Stockholm, Sweden; Department of Advanced Biomedical Sciences, University of Naples Federico II, Naples, Italy

EDUARDO BOSSONE, MD, PhD, FCCP, FESC, FACC
Department of Public Health, Department of Internal Medicine, Interdepartmental Center for Gender Medicine Research (GENESIS), Cardiovascular Disease Fellowship Program, Cardiovascular Pathophysiology and Therapeutics (CardioPath) Ph.D Program, UNESCO Chair on Health Education and Sustainable Development, Faculty of Medicine - University of Naples "Federico II", Italy

YEVGENIY BRAILOVSKY, DO, MSc
Assistant Professor, Department of Advanced Heart Failure and Transplantation, Thomas Jefferson University Hospital, Philadelphia, Pennsylvania, USA

FILIPPO CADEMARTIRI, MD, PhD
Chairman, Department of Imaging, Fondazione Monasterio/CNR, Pisa, Italy

ANDREINA CARBONE, MD
Cardiologist, Department of Internal Medicine, Geriatrics and Neurology, Cardiology Unit, University of Campania Luigi Vanvitelli, Department of Public Health, University of Naples "Federico II", Naples, Italy

THOMAS M. CASCINO, MD, MSc
Clinical Instructor, Division of Cardiology (Frankel Cardiovascular Center), Department of Internal Medicine, University of Michigan, Ann Arbor, Michigan, USA

SAURAV CHATTERJEE, MD
Clinical Assistant Professor, Division of Cardiovascular Medicine, North Shore-Long Island Jewish Medical Centers, Northwell Health, Donald and Barbara Zucker School of Medicine at Hofstra/Northwell, Hempstead, New York, USA

ANTONIO CITTADINI, MD
Full Professor of Internal Medicine, Division of Internal Medicine and Metabolism and Rehabilitation, Department of Translational Medical Sciences, Director, Department of Internal Medicine and Clinical Complexity, University of Naples Federico II, Naples, Italy

WILLIAM K. CORNWELL III, MD, MSCS
Associate Professor, Department of Medicine-Cardiology, Clinical Translational Research Center, University of Colorado Anschutz Medical Campus, Aurora, Colorado, USA

NAGA DHARMAVARAM, MD
Internist, Division of Cardiology, Department of Medicine, University of Wisconsin-Madison, Madison, Wisconsin, USA

KOSTIANTYN DMYTRIIEV, MD
PhD Student, Division of Pulmonary Medicine, Department of Medicine, University of Alberta, Edmonton, Alberta, Canada

PHILIPP DOUSCHAN, MD, PhD
Assistant Professor, Division of Pulmonology, Ludwig Boltzmann Institute for Lung Vascular Research, Medical University of Graz, Graz, Austria; Universities of Giessen and Marburg Lung Center, Member of the German Center for Lung Research (DZL), Justus-Liebig-University, Giessen, Germany

JUSTIN EDWARD, MD
Cardiologist, Department of Medicine-Cardiology, University of Colorado Anschutz Medical Campus, Aurora; Department of Cardiology, Kaiser Permanente, Denver, Colorado, USA

AMIR ESMAEELI, MD
Internal Medicine Specialist, Division of Cardiology, Department of Medicine, University of Wisconsin-Madison, Madison, Wisconsin, USA

FRANCESCO FERRARA, MD, PhD
Cardiologist, Division of Cardiology, Cava de' Tirreni, Cardio-Thoracic-Vascular Department, University Hospital of Salerno, Salerno, Italy

LINDSEY FORBES, MD
Pulmonologist, Division of Pulmonary and Critical Care Medicine, Department of Medicine, University of Colorado Anschutz Medical Campus, Aurora, Colorado, USA

FEDERICA GIARDINO, MD
PhD Fellow, Cardiovascular Pathophysiology and Therapeutics (CardioPath) Program, Internal Medicine Senior Resident, Division of Internal Medicine and Metabolism and Rehabilitation, Department of Translational Medical Sciences, University of Naples Federico II, Naples, Italy

JONATHAN W. HAFT, MD
Professor, Department of Cardiac Surgery, University of Michigan, Ann Arbor, Michigan, USA

TAKENORI IKOMA, MD, PhD
Postdoctoral Research Fellow, Cardiology Division, Cardiovascular Research Center, Massachusetts General Hospital, Boston, Massachusetts, USA

KURT JACOBSON, MD
Interventional Cardiologist, Division of Cardiology, Department of Medicine, University of Wisconsin-Madison, Madison, Wisconsin, USA

ISABELA LANDSTEINER, MD
Postdoctoral Research Fellow, Cardiology Division, Cardiovascular Research Center, Massachusetts General Hospital, Boston, Massachusetts, USA

GREGORY D. LEWIS, MD
Director of Cardiopulmonary Exercise Testing, Cardiology Division, Cardiovascular Research Center, Massachusetts General Hospital, Boston, Massachusetts, USA

BRADLEY A. MARON, MD
Director, Pulmonary Hypertension Center, University of Maryland Medical Center, Senior Associate Dean of Precision Medicine, Department of Medicine, University of Maryland School of Medicine, The University of Maryland-Institute for Health Computing, Baltimore, Maryland, USA

ALBERTO MARIA MARRA, MD, PhD, FEFIM (hon)
Associate Professor of Internal Medicine, Division of Internal Medicine and Metabolism and Rehabilitation, Department of Translational Medical Sciences, University of Naples Federico II, Naples, Italy

ALEXANDRIA MILLER, MD
Assistant Professor of Medicine, Department of Cardiology, The Ohio State University Wexner Medical Center, Davis Heart and Lung Research Institute, Columbus, Ohio, USA

VICTOR M. MOLES, MD
Clinical Assistant Professor, Division of Cardiology (Frankel Cardiovascular Center), Department of Internal Medicine, University of Michigan, Ann Arbor, Michigan, USA

FRANCESCA MUSELLA, MD, PhD
Cardiology Consultant, Cardiology Department, Santa Maria delle Grazie Hospital, Pozzuoli, Naples, Italy; Division of Cardiology, Department of Medicine, Karolinska Institutet, K2 Medicin, Solna, Stockholm, Sweden

STEFANIA PAOLILLO, MD, PhD
Associate Professor of Cardiology, Department of Advanced Biomedical Sciences, University of Naples Federico II, Naples, Italy

HUGH PARKER, MD
Assistant Professor, Department of Medicine-Cardiology, University of Colorado Anschutz Medical Campus, Aurora, Colorado, USA

MARIA VINCENZA POLITO, MD
Cardiologist, Division of Cardiology, Cava de' Tirreni, Cardio-Thoracic-Vascular Department, University Hospital of Salerno, Salerno, Italy

FARHAN RAZA, MD
Assistant Professor, Division of Cardiology, Department of Medicine, University of Wisconsin-Madison, Madison, Wisconsin, USA

MICHAEL G. RISBANO, MD, MA
Division of Pulmonary, Allergy, and Critical Care Medicine, Department of Medicine, Medical Director, Post-COVID Recovery Clinic, University of Pittsburgh School of Medicine and UPMC, Center for Pulmonary Vascular Biology and Medicine, Pittsburgh Heart, Lung, Blood Vascular Medicine Institute, Assistant Professor, Division of Pulmonary, Allergy, Critical Care and Sleep Medicine, Department of Medicine, Vascular Medicine Institute, University of Pittsburgh Medical Center, Montefiore Hospital, Pittsburgh, Pennsylvania, USA

DREW RUBICK, BS
Medical Student, Central Michigan University College of Medical School, Mount Pleasant, Michigan, USA

ERIC RUDOFKER, MD
Internist, Department of Medicine-Cardiology, University of Colorado Anschutz Medical Campus, Aurora, Colorado, USA

SATYAM SARMA, MD
Associate Professor, Department of Internal Medicine, University of Texas Southwestern Medical Center, Institute for Exercise and Environmental Medicine, Texas Health Presbyterian Hospital Dallas, Dallas, Texas, USA

CRISTINA SASSO, MD
Medical Doctor, Department of Medicine,
Surgery and Dentistry, University of Salerno,
Baronissi, Salerno, Italy

MICHAEL K. STICKLAND, PhD
Professor, Division of Pulmonary Medicine,
Department of Medicine, University of Alberta,
G.F. MacDonald Centre for Lung Health,
Covenant Health, Edmonton, Alberta,
Canada

EMMETT SUCKOW, BS
Clinical Trial Coordinator, Department of
Medicine-Cardiology, University of Colorado
Anschutz Medical Campus, Aurora, Colorado,
USA

NATALIE VAN OCHTEN, MD
Resident Physician, Department of Medicine,
University of Colorado Anschutz Medical
Campus, Aurora, Colorado, USA

GABRIELLA VANAKEN, MD
Internal Medicine Resident, University of
Michigan Medical School, Department of
Internal Medicine, University of Michigan, Ann
Arbor, Michigan, USA

REBECCA R. VANDERPOOL, PhD
Assistant Professor, Division of Cardiovascular
Medicine, The Ohio State University Wexner
Medical Center, Davis Heart and Lung
Research Institute, Columbus, Ohio, USA

SCOTT H. VISOVATTI, MD, FACC, FCCP
Director, Pulmonary Hypertension and
Pulmonary Embolism Program, Clinical
Associate Professor, Division of
Cardiovascular Medicine, Department of
Internal Medicine, The Ohio State University
College of Medicine, Columbus, Ohio, USA

JASON WEATHERALD, MD, MSc
Associate Professor, Division of Pulmonary
Medicine, Department of Medicine, University
of Alberta, Edmonton, Alberta, Canada

DANIEL WIECZOREK, BS
Medical Student, University of Michigan
Medical School, Ann Arbor, Michigan, USA

KYLA WULFF, BSN, RN
Registered Nurse, Clinical Translational
Research Center, University of Colorado
Anschutz Medical Campus, Aurora, Colorado,
USA

Contents

Pulmonary arterial hypertension (PAH) is a progressive pulmonary vascular disease that has a high impact on patients' quality of life, morbidity and mortality. PAH is characterized by extensive pulmonary vascular remodeling that results in an increase in pulmonary vascular resistance and right ventricular afterload, and can lead to right heart failure. Patients with PAH exhibit inefficient ventilation, high dead space ventilation, dynamic hyperinflation, and ventricular-arterial uncoupling, which can contribute to high dyspnea and low exercise tolerance. Cardiopulmonary exercise testing can help to diagnose PAH, define prognosis and treatment response in PAH, as well as discriminate between different pulmonary vascular diseases.

The pulmonary circulation and the right ventricle play a pivotal role in the global hemodynamics of human beings, so much so that their close interaction is encapsulated in the concept of a "morpho-functional unit". In this review we aim to pinpoint the strengths and weaknesses of various noninvasive established techniques. The goal is to detect early morphologic and/or functional changes in the pulmonary circulation and right ventricular unit, which is crucial for tailoring treatments and prognostic assessments. The scope of this review includes resting and stress echocardiography, cardiopulmonary exercise testing, computed tomography, and cardiac magnetic resonance in characterizing the pulmonary circulation-right ventricular unit both morphologically and functionally.

The invasive cardiopulmonary exercise test (iCPET) provides a comprehensive, simultaneous evaluation of an individual's cardiovascular, respiratory, and metabolic response to exercise. The test is uniquely suited for the evaluation of exercise intolerance, as well as the deep phenotyping of disease states including pulmonary arterial hypertension and post–coronavirus disease symptomatology. Despite an expanding list of clinical and research applications, both the complexity of the test and a lack of familiarity with how the test is performed have been barriers to the widespread use of iCPET. The aim of this article is to provide practical insights into how an iCPET is performed.

Invasive cardiopulmonary exercise testing (iCPET) is increasingly recognized as a critical diagnostic tool for assessing exercise intolerance and dyspnea. The manuscript highlights the iCPET program's diagnostic precision in identifying various cardiopulmonary disorders, offering insights into tailored treatment strategies. This guide aims to assist institutions in establishing their iCPET programs, addressing both the technical and administrative facets essential for success. The narrative is rooted in personal experiences, reflecting on the demanding, yet rewarding, journey of enhancing patient care through advanced diagnostic capabilities.

Cardiopulmonary exercise testing is an active research area in patients with unexplained dyspnea, heart failure, and pulmonary hypertension. Focus has centered on the use of novel hemodynamic parameters to further characterize these disease states, influence therapeutics, and determine prognosis. Translational research focuses on the underlying cardiopulmonary physiology to more precisely quantify the effect of pulmonary vascular disease on the right ventricle and pulmonary function/hemodynamics. In addition, phenotyping unexplained dyspnea is of critical importance, given the significant heterogeneity of this patient population with implications for therapies and clinical trial design.

Long-term exercise intolerance and functional limitations are common after an episode of acute pulmonary embolism (PE), despite 3 to 6 months of anticoagulation. These persistent symptoms are reported in more than half of the patients with acute PE and are referred as "post-PE syndrome." Although these functional limitations can occur from persistent pulmonary vascular occlusion or pulmonary vascular remodeling, significant deconditioning can be a major contributing factor. Herein, the authors review the role of exercise testing to elucidate the mechanisms of exercise limitations to guide next steps in management and exercise training for musculoskeletal deconditioning.

Of the 5 randomized controlled trials (RCTs) included, chronic thromboembolic pulmonary hypertension (CTEPH) patients constituted 20% of the overall pulmonary hypertension (PH) patient population. We did not find any RCTs that evaluated the role of exercise training in patients with CTEPH. The results of this study indicate that exercise training may be effective at improving exercise capacity, as measured by 6-min walk distance, in patients with PH. Another notable finding from this analysis is the lack of adverse events associated with exercise training, suggesting that contrary to widespread perception, exercise training is safe in CTEPH and PAH patients.

HEART FAILURE CLINICS

FORTHCOMING ISSUES

RECENT ISSUES

SERIES OF RELATED INTEREST

Cardiology Clinics
http://www.cardiology.theclinics.com/
Cardiac Electrophysiology Clinics
https://www.cardiacep.theclinics.com/
Interventional Cardiology Clinics
https://www.interventional.theclinics.com/

THE CLINICS ARE AVAILABLE ONLINE!
Access your subscription at:
www.theclinics.com

Preface

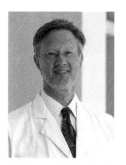

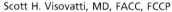

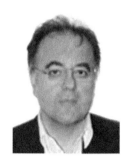

Scott H. Visovatti, MD, FACC, FCCP   Eduardo Bossone, MD, PhD, FCCP, FESC, FACC

Editors

I thought of that while riding my bike.
—Albert Einstein on the Theory of Relativity

As this quote by Albert Einstein reminds us, exercise can lead to great understanding. In this special issue of *Heart Failure Clinics*, we discuss the breakthroughs in our understanding of heart failure and pulmonary hypertension that have been made possible through exercise testing. In addition, we explore the role of exercise in the evaluation and treatment of patients with these conditions. Recognizing and interpreting abnormal responses to exercise in disease states is possible only after first becoming familiar with normal responses. Thus, the discussion begins with Ferrara and colleagues' enlightening review of invasive and noninvasive means of monitoring the right-heart–pulmonary circulation unit's response to exercise in healthy individuals. Rudifker and colleagues then take us to one extreme in the spectrum of health in their insightful overview of the responses to exercise in elite athletes.

Next, we explore the value of exercise testing in the evaluation of patients with diseases, including heart failure or pulmonary hypertension. The maximal oxygen uptake (vo_2max) during noninvasive cardiopulmonary exercise testing (CPET) has a well-established role in the assessment of prognosis, response to therapy, and candidacy for advanced therapies in patients with heart failure with reduced ejection fraction. In his contribution, Sarma provides fresh insight into diagnostic and prognostic applications of exercise hemodynamics in heart failure with preserved ejection fraction; he also addressed challenges associated with performing and interpreting exercise studies.

As shown in the elegant contribution from Dmytriiev and colleagues, exercise testing also plays an important role in diagnosis, phenotyping, and treatment response assessment in patients with pulmonary vascular disease. Giardino and colleagues delve even further into the use of noninvasive exercise testing in the assessment of pulmonary vascular disease in their innovative investigation that focuses on the pulmonary circulation–right-ventricular functional unit. Switching to an invasive exercise testing option for the diagnosis of cardiopulmonary disease, we take a deep dive into the invasive cardiopulmonary exercise test (iCPET). This test provides an assessment of an individual's hemodynamic, ventilatory, and gas exchange responses to exercise by combining CPET with exercise right-heart catheterization. While unique in its ability to provide a comprehensive evaluation of an individual's response to exercise, the test's complexity and a general lack of familiarity with how it is performed have resulted in underuse of iCPET. To help strike down these barriers to widespread use of iCPET, we provide companion contributions: Visovatti and colleague present an in-depth, practical description of how to set up and perform the test, and Risbano provides an accessible, all-inclusive discussion on how to establish an iCPET program.

Heart Failure Clin 21 (2025) xi–xii
https://doi.org/10.1016/j.hfc.2024.09.009
1551-7136/25/© 2024 Published by Elsevier Inc.

The rapid expansion of exercise testing in the clinical arena is mirrored by impressive growth in research applications. Miller and colleague provide an exciting overview of the current state of how exercise testing is currently being used in research studies, as well as future directions for growth.

Just as exciting as the expanding roles of diagnostic exercise testing in heart failure and pulmonary hypertension is our growing understanding of exercise as therapy. We present two articles addressing the use of exercise in patients with persistent functional intolerance following pulmonary embolism. Dharmavaram and colleagues provide an excellent overview of the use of use of exercise testing in the evaluation and treatment of cardiopulmonary diseases (including chronic thromboembolic pulmonary hypertension [CTEPH]). Van Aken and colleagues present a meta-analysis of randomized controlled trials suggesting that exercise training is safe and effective in CTEPH patients.

What is next for exercise testing? Clinical trials, real-world evidence, and our daily clinical experiences have made us aware of the need for ever-deepening phenotyping in order to more fully understand these complex conditions and tailor therapies. Long gone are classification systems based upon broad concepts, such as primary versus secondary pulmonary hypertension. Instead, the recent 2022 European Society of Cardiology/European Respiratory Society Guidelines for the diagnosis and treatment of pulmonary hypertension classifies pulmonary hypertension into five different groups based upon similar pathophysiologic mechanisms, clinical characteristics, hemodynamic patterns, and therapeutic management.[1] Similarly, what was once known as "heart failure" has been further subclassified, including a four-subgroup system based upon ejection fraction.[2] We believe that exercise testing will play an essential role in even deeper phenotyping and subclassification of heart failure and pulmonary hypertension, creating opportunity for a better understanding of these diseases and more tailored therapeutic approaches.

In conclusion, this special issue of *Heart Failure Clinics* provides insight into the expanding roles of exercise in the evaluation and treatment of pulmonary hypertension and heart failure. I am grateful to the authors for their contributions on this important topic.

DISCLOSURES

The authors have no conflicts of interest to disclose.

Scott H. Visovatti, MD, FACC, FCCP
Division of Cardiovascular Medicine
The Ohio State University
Pulmonary Hypertension and
Pulmonary Embolism Program
Columbus, OH, USA

Eduardo Bossone, MD, PhD, FCCP, FESC, FACC
Department of Public Health
Department of Internal Medicine
Interdepartmental Center for
Gender Medicine Research (GENESIS)
Cardiovascular Disease Fellowship Program
Cardiovascular Pathophysiology and
Therapeutics (CardioPath) Ph.D Program
UNESCO Chair on Health
Education and Sustainable Development
Faculty of Medicine - University of Naples
"Federico II", Italy

Ed. 18, I piano
Via Sergio Pansini 5
80131 – Naples, Italy

E-mail addresses:
Scott.visovatti@osumc.edu (S.H. Visovatti)
eduardo.bossone@unina.it (E. Bossone)

REFERENCES

1. Humbert M, Kovacs G, Hoeper MM, et al. 2022 ESC/ERS guidelines for the diagnosis and treatment of pulmonary hypertension. Eur Heart J 2022;43(38):3618–731.
2. Heidenreich PA, Bozkurt B, Aguilar D, et al. 2022 AHA/ACC/HFSA guideline for the management of heart failure: executive summary: a report of the American College of Cardiology/American Heart Association Joint Committee on clinical practice guidelines. J Am Coll Cardiol 2022;79(17):1757–80.

Normal Hemodynamic Response to Exercise

Francesco Ferrara, MD, PhD[a,1], Andreina Carbone, MD[b,c,1], Maria Vincenza Polito, MD[a], Cristina Sasso, MD[d], Eduardo Bossone, MD, PhD[e,1,*]

KEYWORDS

- Right heart • Pulmonary circulation • Pulmonary hypertension • Exercise right-heart catheterization
- Exercise Doppler echocardiography

KEY POINTS

- Exercise stress measurements of the pulmonary circulation may detect early stage pulmonary vascular and/or left heart diseases.
- Pulmonary vascular pressures are flow-dependent with invasively determined upper limits of normal for mean pulmonary artery pressure (mPAP) and pulmonary artery wedge pressure (PAWP) as a function of cardiac output (CO)relationships of 3 mm Hg/L/min and 2 mm Hg/L/min, respectively.
- Among non-invasive methods, exercise transthoracic echocardiography (TTE) is the most widely available and sustainable.
- The RIGHT heart international NETwork ("RIGHT-NET") meta-model for the study of the right heart pulmonary circulation unit provided standardization of exercise TTE through a robust methodological approach. An upper limit of normal mPAP/CO slope was found at 3.5 mm Hg/L/min, slightly higher than reported invasive cut-off values.

INTRODUCTION

During the last years, there has been an increased awareness of the importance of exercise stress measurements of the pulmonary circulation to detect early stage pulmonary vascular and/or left heart diseases (PVD, LHD).[1] In this regard, the 2022 European Society of Cardiology/European Respiratory Society (ESC/ERS) Guidelines for the diagnosis and treatment of pulmonary hypertension (PH) reintroduced the hemodynamic definition of exercise PH as an invasive mean pulmonary artery pressure (mPAP)/cardiac output (CO) slope greater than 3 mm Hg/L/min between rest and exercise.[2] However, the real clinical relevance of abnormal responses in subjects at risk or with overt PH remains unclear. Herein, the authors review the invasive versus non-invasive monitoring of the right heart-pulmonary circulation unit (RH-PCU) response to exercise in healthy subjects.

[a] Division of Cardiology, Cava de' Tirreni, Cardio-Thoracic-Vascular Department, University Hospital of Salerno, Via Enrico de Marinis, 84013 Cava de' Tirreni - SA, Italy; [b] Department of Internal Medicine, Geriatrics and Neurology, Cardiology Unit, University of Campania Luigi Vanvitelli, Naples 80138, Italy; [c] Department of Public Health, University of Naples "Federico II", Via Pansini, 5, Naples 80131, Italy; [d] Department of Medicine, Surgery and Dentistry, University of Salerno, Via Salvador Allende, 43, 84081, Baronissi, Salerno, Italy; [e] Department of Public Health Department of Internal Medicine Interdepartmental Center for Gender Medicine Research (GENESIS) Cardiovascular Disease Fellowship Program Cardiovascular Pathophysiology and Therapeutics (CardioPath) Ph.D Program UNESCO Chair on Health Education and Sustainable Development Faculty of Medicine - University of Naples "Federico II", Ed. 18, I piano, Via Sergio Pansini 5, 80131 – Naples, Italy
[1] These authors contributed equally.
* Corresponding author. Department of Public Health University of Naples "Federico II", Via Pansini, 5, 80131, Naples, Italy.
E-mail address: eduardo.bossone@unina.it

Heart Failure Clin 21 (2025) 1–14
https://doi.org/10.1016/j.hfc.2024.06.001
1551-7136/25/© 2024 Elsevier Inc. All rights are reserved, including those for text and data mining, AI training, and similar technologies.

heartfailure.theclinics.com

PHYSIOLOGIC PULMONARY CIRCULATION RESPONSE TO EXERCISE

The RH-PCU is an anatomic and functional complex system characterized by high flow, low pressure, and low resistance.[3] Accordingly, the Poiseuille-Hagen equation, extrapolated to pulmonary circulation, states pulmonary vascular resistance (PVR) = [pulmonary artery pressure (PAP) - left atrial pressure (LAP)]/CO and may be rewritten as mPAP = PVR × CO + pulmonary artery wedge pressure (PAWP).

In normal conditions, exercise results in major increases in pulmonary flow (CO can increase 2.5 up to 10 times during exercise) and minor changes in pulmonary pressures. In general, the mPAP-CO relationship may be better described by a linear approximation, where (on average) each liter per minute of increase in CO is accompanied by an increase of 1 mm Hg in mPAP in a young adult (Fig. 1).[4] The mPAP/CO slope is steeper in older healthy subjects of 60 to 80 years, and compared to young individuals the same increase in CO is accompanied by a 2-3 fold higher rise in pulmonary pressures. However, since there is a large individual variation, the best method for a definition of limits of normal would be to adjust multipoint PAP-CO relationships for individual variability, as reported in noninvasive studies.[5] Exercise PH is defined by a mPAP normal at rest but greater than 30 mm Hg during exercise at a cardiac output less than 10 L/min, or mPAP-CO greater than 3 mm Hg/L/min (see Fig. 1; Fig. 2).[2,6–8] In several diseases, determining abnormal right heart loading conditions through different pathophysiologic pathways, may lead to a pathologic increase of pulmonary pressures first during exercise (early-stage disease) and only later at rest (advanced disease).[9]

In this regard, pulmonary pressures may abnormally increase in the presence of (a) increased PVR due to PVD (eg, pulmonary arterial hypertension, congenital heart disease, portal hypertension, hypoxia, lung disease, pulmonary embolism, other unknow mechanisms); (b) elevated pulmonary blood flow (eg, liver disease, hyperthyroidism, and sickle cell disease); (c) increased PAWP due to any cause of LHD (heart failure, coronary artery disease, cardiomyopathies, valve disease, etc.).[2] The measurement of exercise PAWP is crucial to differentiate pre-capillary versus post-capillary PH. Likewise, for mPAP, PAWP increases as a function of CO during exercise. A 3-fold increase in CO with minor increase in PAWP occurs in healthy subjects, while the same increase in CO determines a steep rise in PAWP and extravascular lung water in heart failure patients. The Invasive PAWP-CO relationship has been shown to increase by an average of 1 mm Hg/L/min,[4] and remains below 2 mm Hg/L/min, in healthy subjects.[6]

Of note, in elite athletes, the observed exercise-induced increase in pulmonary pressure is a "physiologic phenomenon" directly related to supernormal flow, resulting in a mild increase in left ventricular (LV) filling pressure and a slight decreased PVR.[10] At extreme levels of exercise, a significant rise in the LV filling pressure my occur, resulting in stress failure of pulmonary capillaries and related exercise-induced pulmonary hemorrhage; this response has been seen in racehorses.[11]

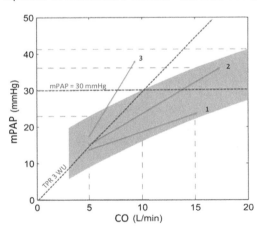

Fig. 1. Mean pulmonary artery pressure (mPAP) as a function of cardiac output (CO) in 3 subjects (arrows): The subjects 1 and 2 are normal, even though the subject 2 has an exercise mPAP greater than 30 mm Hg, and the subject 3 has an abnormal response suggesting exercise pulmonary hypertension. A prediction band defining limits of normal (shaded area) was calculated by quadratic fitting of pooled pressure-flow data from 137 healthy volunteers reported in Lewis and colleagues.[6] TPR, total pulmonary resistance; WU, Wood units. (Reprinted with permission from Lewis GD, Bossone E, Naeije R, et al. Pulmonary vascular hemodynamic response to exercise in cardiopulmonary diseases. Circulation 2013;128:1470-79.[7])

INVASIVE VERSUS NON-INVASIVE MONITORING OF THE RIGHT HEART AND PULMONARY CIRCULATION UNIT RESPONSE TO EXERCISE
Right Heart Catheterization

Right heart catheterization (RHC) is the gold standard test to assess resting and exercise pulmonary hemodynamics. Some practical issues have been addressed by the official European Respiratory Society statement on pulmonary hemodynamics during exercise[12]: (a) the zero reference level must be set at the left atrial level (midthoracic level in the supine position) for both rest and exercise; (b) systolic and diastolic pulmonary pressures may be better assessed by micromanometer-tipped catheter

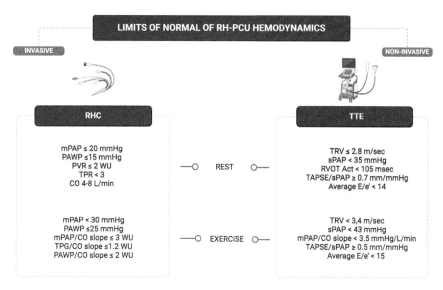

Fig. 2. Invasive versus non-invasive limits of normal of right heart and pulmonary circulation hemodynamics.[2,6,20,26,27,39] CO, cardiac output; mPAP, mean pulmonary artery pressure; PAWP, pulmonary artery wedge pressure; PVR, pulmonary vascular resistance; RHC, right heart catheterization; RH-PCU, right heart-pulmonary circulation unit; RVOT, right ventricle outflow tract; sPAP, systolic pulmonary artery pressure; TAPSE, tricuspid annular plane systolic excursion; TPG, transpulmonary pressure gradient; TPR, total peripheral resistance; WU, Wood units; TTE, transthoracic echocardiography.

because of aliasing artifacts with fluid-filled catheter; (c) the direct Fick principle is the gold standard for determination of CO, based on the principle that oxygen consumption (Vo_2) is equal to the product of the blood flow to the peripheral tissues and the arterial-venous oxygen concentration difference. Vo_2 must be directly measured and not taken from tables relying on standardized resting conditions in healthy subjects; (d) incremental exercise tests (step or ramp protocol) must to be used, avoiding prolonged and isometric exercise tests; (e) a venous approach via the jugular or the cubital vein for the insertion of the pulmonary artery should be preferred in exercise studies with cycle ergometry; (f) repeated hemodynamic measurements, systemic and pulmonary arterial blood gas analysis should be performed at least at rest and at peak exercise; (e) averaging vascular pressures over several respiratory cycles should be preferred instead of reading them at end-expiration in order to avoid the influence of negative inspiratory and positive expiratory pleural pressures.[12]

Although a low incidence of complications are reported, the risk/benefit ratio of the invasive assessment of pulmonary hemodynamics during exercise may be unfavorable and/or unjustifiable in the following conditions: (a) healthy controls; (b) patients who did not undergo a thorough diagnostic work-up at rest; (c) patients with unstable disease or decompensated RH failure. Essential measurements and calculations during exercise are mPAP, PAWP and

CO, derived total pulmonary resistance (TPR) (mPAP/CO), and PVR ((mPAP − PAWP)/CO) as well as the mPAP/CO and PAWP/CO slopes.[12] However, CO measurements during exercise may be challenging. Workload and Vo_2 may be used as surrogates to CO, as they are linearly related (when CO is not too high), In this regard, the following linear regression equations to predict CO during exercise in healthy volunteers may be used[13]:

CO (L/min) = 0.34 × Vo_2 (mL/kg/min) + 5.4.
CO (L = min) = 0.06 workload (W) + 6.5.

However, significant interindividual variability of these relationships alter the reliability of the prediction and the estimation of CO; therefore, these variables are not interchangeable.[8]

Furthermore, the assessment of PAWP may be technically challenging, especially during exercise. A common pitfall is an under-wedged (incompletely occluded) pulmonary artery that may lead to an overestimation of true PAWP due to a hybrid measurement of both left atrial and pulmonary artery pressures.[12] Different exercise protocols and body position (semi-upright, supine, and semi-supine) have been reported among highly specialized expert centers.[6,14]

An overview of exercise RHC studies for the evaluation of the RH-PCU in healthy subjects (sample size > 20 subjects), published after 2003, is reported in **Table 1**.[15–18] Invasively determined mPAP-CO and PAWP-CO relationships during exercise have been reported in sufficiently-size cohorts of healthy

Table 1
Overview of the invasive published studies for evaluation of the pulmonary and left heart pressure in healthy subjects

Study	N	Age (y)	Exercise Level	Body Position During Exercise	Resting HR (bpm)	Exercise HR (bpm)	Resting mPAP (mm Hg)	Exercise mPAP (mm Hg)	Resting PAWP (mm Hg)	Exercise PAWP (mm Hg)	Resting PVR/PVRI (WU)	Exercise PVR/PVRI (WU)	Resting CI (L/min/m2)	Exercise CI (L/min/m2)	Resting CO (L/min)	Exercise CO (L/min)	Watt
Wright et al,[15] 2016	28	55 ± 6	Moderate and light exercise levels	Semi-UP	63 ± 8	122 ± 2	17 ± 3	25 ± 6	11 ± 3	15 ± 5	1.28 ± 0.39	0.96 ± 0.38	-	6.8 ± 1.5	4.8 ± 0.8	11.1 ± 2.8	-
Esfandiari et al,[16] 2017	18	58 ± 6	Moderate and light exercise levels	Semi-UP	64 ± 8	122 ± 3	18 ± 2	26 ± 6	12 ± 2	15 ± 5	1.49 ± 0.61	1.2 ± 0.3	2.5 ± 0.4	5.4 ± 1.8	4.6 ± 0.6	10.3 ± 1.5	-
Esfandiari et al,[16] 2017	18	54 ± 7	Moderate and light exercise levels	Semi-UP	62 ± 7	121 ± 2	17 ± 3	25 ± 6	11 ± 3	15 ± 5	1.3 ± 0.4	1.14 ± 0.4	2.8 ± 0.6	6.6 ± 1.9	5.1 ± 0.9	12.3 ± 3.2	-
Wolsk et al,[17] 2017	20	29 (20–39)	Individual peak, moderate and light exercise	SUP	63 (95% CI 57–69)	141 (95% CI 132–151)	13 (95% CI 12–14)	25 (95% CI 22–28)	9 (95% CI 8–9)	13 (95% CI 10–15)	0.8 (IQR 0.7–1)	0.7 (95% CI 0.6–0.8)	2.9 (95% CI 2.6–3.1)	9.9 (95% CI 9.6–10.4)	-	-	174 (95% CI 155–192)
Wolsk et al,[17] 2017	22	49 (40–59)	Individual peak, moderate and light exercise	SUP	64 (95% CI 60–69)	126 (95% CI 117–135)	15 (95% CI 13–16)	32 (95% CI 27–38)	9 (95% CI 8–10)	19 (95% CI 15–23)	1 (IQR 0.8–1.2)	0.8 (95% CI 0.8–1)	2.8 (95% CI 2.6–2.9)	8.8 (95% CI 8.4–9.3)	-	-	144 (95% CI 129–159)

Study	n	Age	Exercise level	Position													
Wolsk et al,[17] 2017	20	69 (60–80)	Peak, moderate and light exercise level	SUP	62 (95% CI 58–66)	128 (95% CI 121–136)	15 (95% CI 14–16)	39 (95% CI 36–43)	8 (95% CI 7–9)	23 (95% CI 21–25)	1.5 (IQR 1.2–1.7)	1.1 (95% CI 0.9–1.4)	2.6 (95% CI 2.4–2.8)	7.9 (95% CI 7.2–8.6)	-	130 (95% CI 113–147)	
Andersen et al,[18] 2019	16	31 (18–40)	Individual peak	Semi-SUP[a]	62 ± 13	145 ± 17	12 ± 3	23 ± 5	8 ± 2	13 ± 4	0.7 ± 0.3	0.6 ± 0.1	2.9 ± 0.4	10 ± 0.8	5.5 ± 1.1	18.8 ± 1.7	-
Andersen et al,[18] 2019	15	49 (40–59)	Individual peak	Semi-SUP[a]	66 ± 9	138 ± 14	14 ± 3	31 ± 12	9 ± 3	19 ± 10	0.9 ± 0.3	0.7 ± 0.4	2.7 ± 0.3	9.1 ± 1.3	5.1 ± 0.9	17.1 ± 2.6	-
Andersen et al,[18] 2019	19	69 (60–80)	Individual peak	Semi-SUP[a]	63 ± 8	129 ± 16	14 ± 3	36 ± 7	8 ± 3	23 ± 5	1.3 ± 0.5	0.9 ± 0.3	2.6 ± 0.4	7.9 ± 1.3	5 ± 1	14.7 ± 2.8	-

Data are presented as mean ± standard deviation (SD) or median (IQR). 95% CI: 95% confidence interval. Exercise protocol was ergometry for all studies.

Abbreviations: bpm: beats per minute; CI, cardiac index; CO, cardiac output; HR, heart rate; L, liter; min: minute; mPAP, mean pulmonary arterial pressure; PAWP, pulmonary arterial wedge pressure; PVR, pulmonary vascular resistance; PVRI, pulmonary vascular resistance index; Semi-SUP, semi-supine; Semi-UP, semi-upright; SUP, supine; WU, wood units.

a Body position is different at rest.

volunteers (n = 250 subjects from 11 studies).[6] In the supine position, mPAP (13.5 ± 2.0 vs 29.2 ± 5.3 mm Hg) and PAWP (8.6 ± 0.6 vs 17.8 ± 3.7 mm Hg) increased significantly during exercise, while PVR (1.0 ± 0.2 vs 0.8 ± 0.2WU) showed a trend for a slight decrease.[6] Various cut-offs from 20 to 25 mm Hg have been considered as the upper limit of normal for PAWP during exercise (see **Fig. 2**).[19,20] In this regard, an invasive hemodynamic peak PAWP ≥ 25 mm Hg during exercise in the supine position allowed diagnosis of heart failure preserved ejection fraction (HFpEF) in patients with exertional dyspnea, normal ejection fraction, and resting PAWP ≤ 15 mm Hg, according to the European Society of Cardiology (ESC) diagnostic algorithm for HFpEF.[20] However, invasive hemodynamic variables addressing the pressure-flow relationship, namely mPAP/CO, PAWP/CO, and trans-pulmonary gradient (TPG)/CO slopes, might better characterize left and right hemodynamic during exercise.[6,21] Notably, both mPAP/CO slope and PAWP/CO slope are strongly age-dependent. The upper limit of normal (ULN) of mPAP/CO slope (supine position) ranges from 1.6 Wood units (WU) (in ∼30-year-old healthy subjects) to 3.3 WU (in ∼70-year-old healthy subjects).[4,6] These findings suggest that the aging process is related to a reduction of pulmonary vascular and LV compliance.[22] Accordingly, 2022 ESC/ERS PH Guidelines revised definition of exercise PH as an invasively assessed

mPAP-CO greater than 3 mm Hg/L/min. A PAWP/CO slope greater than 2 mm Hg/L/min may be useful to differentiate post-capillary versus pre-capillary causes of exercise PH (see **Fig. 2**).[23] The ULN of TPG/CO slope is 1.2 WU and this variable appears to be age-independent. It should be underlined that resting and exercise PAWP thresholds alone might be insufficient to differentiate pre-capillary from post-capillary PH, and should be considered in the clinical context of the patient (phenotype, risk factors) and echocardiographic findings, including left heart structure and function.

Exercise Transthoracic Doppler Echocardiography

Among non-invasive exercise methods (TTE, cardiopulmonary test, cardiac magnetic resonance) for the study of the RH-PCU, exercise TTE is the most widely available and sustainable (**Fig. 3**).[24–26] TTE provides comprehensive information on right and left heart morphology and function, along with estimates of resting and exercise hemodynamic parameters (**Fig. 4**). Although the diagnosis of exercise PH still relies on invasive measurements, substantial data suggest that exercise TTE may be sufficient to unmask early abnormalities of the pulmonary vascular bed.[26]

Exercise TTE measurements of the RH-PCU appear to agree very well with those obtained during RHC.[27,28] In this regard, echocardiographic estimates of PAP from the tricuspid regurgitation

Test	Availability	Invasiveness	Anatomy	RV function	Hemodinamic information	Prognostic information	Accuracy	Radiation exposure (mSV)	Carbon cost (CO₂ kg)	Costs	Sustainability[a]
Exercise RHC	++	+++	++	+	++++	+++	++++	High	C C	€ €	✿ ✿
Exercise TTE	+++	+	+++	+++	++	++	+++	No	C	€	✿ ✿ ✿
Cardiopulmonary exercise	+++	+	+	+	+	++	+	No	C	€	✿
Exercise CMR	++	+	++++	++++	+	+	++	No	C C C	€ €	✿
Exercise CMR with simultaneous invasive pressure registration	+	+++	++++	++++	++++	+	++++	High	C C C	€ € €	✿

Fig. 3. Comparison between different exercise tests for the assessment of the right heart-pulmonary circulation Unit. +: scarse; ++: reasonable; +++: good; ++++: optimal; CMR, cardiac magnetic resonance; RHC, right heart catheterization; TTE, transthoracic echocardiography. Radiation exposure expressed as effective dose in milliSievert (mSV) per examination: High (about 7 mSV). Carbon cost expressed in kg of carbon dioxide (CO_2) emissions per examination: Low (2Kg), Medium (10–20Kg), High (200–300 kg). [a]Sustainability Index = Accuracy/k € + mSv + Kg CO_2.[24] The "sustainability index" could be calculated for every diagnostic and medical imaging examination. The numerator is the accuracy, best assessed by the physician. The denominator includes the sum of the direct cost (covered by the payer, in thousands of euros), the long-term radiation risk (in mSv), and the carbon cost (in kg of carbon dioxide emissions). The higher the value, the more sustainable the medical imaging examination.

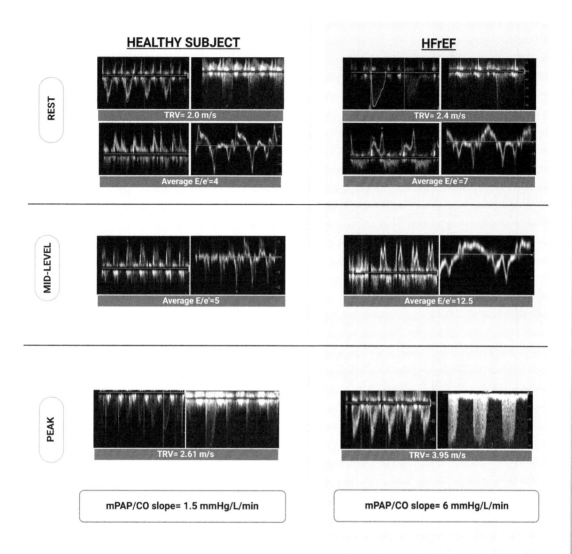

Fig. 4. Right heart pulmonary circulation response during exercise Doppler echocardiography in age-matched healthy subjects versus heart failure patient. A 77-year-old healthy woman without cardiovascular risk factors versus a 77-year-old woman with diagnosis of heart failure (NYHA class III) with reduced ejection fraction (EF 40%). CO, cardiac output; E, peak PW Doppler velocity of mitral inflow; e', average of septal and lateral mitral annular peak tissue Doppler velocities; mPAP, mean pulmonary artery pressure; TRV, tricuspid regurgitant peak velocity.

maximum velocity (TRV), compared to invasively measured PAP during exercise have been shown to have acceptable accuracy (only minimal bias), but limited precision (wide limits of agreement) by Bland & Altman analysis.[29,30] Furthermore, the agreement between TTE and invasive measures of PAP during upright exercise improves among the subset of patients with high-quality TRV Doppler signal.[30] An overview of the main published studies for exercise echocardiography in healthy subjects (>50) is reported in **Table 2**.[31–38] However, concern remains that TTE may underestimate CO during

exercise.[29] This can probably be overcome by intensive training of dedicated operators. In addition, the E/e' ratio demonstrated a good positive predictive value (85%–93%) for diagnosis of elevated exercise PAWP, but the negative predictive value is low (55%–77%), resulting in a substantial false negative results.[39] Recently, Harada and colleagues demonstrated that the cutoff value of E/e' ≤ 12.4 during 20 W exercise may be very accurate at predicting patients with E/e' ratio greater than 15 at peak exercise (specificity = 94%; positive predictive value = 98%). Furthermore, in a subset of

Table 2
Overview of the main published studies for exercise echocardiography in healthy subjects (>50)

Study	N	Age (y)	Height (cm)	Weight (kg)	BMI (kg/m2)	Baseline HR (bpm)	Peak HR (bpm)	Exercise Protocol Workload (W/METs)	RAP Estimate (mm Hg)	Baseline sPAP (mm Hg)	Peak sPAP (mm Hg)	ΔsPAP (mm Hg)	Baseline TRV (m/s)	Peak TRV (m/s)	E/E′ Ratio	Baseline CO (L/min)	Peak CO (L/min)
Grunig et al,[31] 2009	191	32 ± 10	173 ± 9	68 ± 12	-	74 ± 13	-	Supine bicycle (125)	From IVC	20,4 ± 5,3	35,5 ± 5,4	15.2 ± 7.1	1,98 ± 0,31	2,81 ± 0,31	-	-	-
Mahjoub et al,[32] 2009	70	48 ± 16	-	-	24,6 ± 4,2	71 ± 12	-	Semisupine bicycle (152 ± 47)	Fixed value (5)	27 ± 4	51 ± 9	27 ± 8	2,0 ± 0,2	-	7 ± 4	5,0 ± 1,3	-
D'Alto et al,[33] 2011	88	55,3 ± 12,5	161,5 ± 8	64,1 ± 11,3	-	81,1 ± 11,1	126 ± 18	Supine bicycle (89 ± 28)	From IVC	20,6 ± 3,7	25,9 ± 3,3	5,3 ± 4,1	-	-	-	-	-
Argiento et al,[4] 2012	124	37 ± 13	173 ± 9	70 ± 11	-	-	-	Supine bicycle (175 ± 50)	Fixed value (5)	15,5 ± 2,6 M; 15,1 ± 2,9 F	36 ± 5,9 M; 30,5 ± 7,2 F	-	-	-	-	5.9 ± 1.4 M; 4,6 ± 0,8 F	20,5 ± 4,1 M; 14,8 ± 3,2 F
Chia et al,[34] 2015	50	52,9 ± 9,2	164,4 ± 9,5	69,4 ± 10,8	-	74 ± 11	162 ± 14	Treadmill exercise (10,3 ± 3,5)	From IVC	22,7 ± 6,9	29,3 ± 11,8	6,1 ± 9,8	-	-	-	-	-
D'Alto et al,[35] 2017	90	39 ± 13	173 ± 9	70 ± 11	-	72 ± 9	152 ± 16	Semisupine bicycle (177 ± 50)	From IVC	22 ± 5	34 ± 7	12 ± 9	-	-	5,1 ± 3,1	5,1 ± 1,2	18,2 ± 4,2
D'Andrea et al,[36] 2018	50	59,4 ± 6,3	-	-	28,3 ± 2	73,5 ± 8,2	115,3 ± 26	Supine bicycle (125,4 ± 50)	From IVC	15,3 ± 6	32,5 ± 5	16,9 ± 3,3	-	-	6,4 ± 3,1	-	-
Wierzbowska-Drabik et al,[37] 2020	50	52 ± 14	-	-	26,5 ± 4,4	68 ± 13	131 ± 22	Semisupine bicycle (133 ± 42)	From IVC	23 ± 10	32 ± 12	-	2,91 ± 0,51	2,52 ± 0,7	-	4,28 ± 2,3	-
Vriz et al,[38] 2022	145	54 ± 14,9	-	-	26 ± 3,5	75 ± 15	138 ± 18	Semisupine bicycle (133 ± 38)	From IVC	22 ± 3	35,4 ± 9,4	13,6 ± 9,1	-	-	7,3 ± 2,5	5,1 ± 1,7	12,5 ± 3,1

Data are presented as mean ± standard deviation (SD) or median (IQR).
Abbreviations: BMI, body mass index; CI, cardiac index; CO, cardiac output; F, female; M, male; RAP, right atrial pressure; sPAP, systolic pulmonary artery pressure.

KEY METHODOLOGICAL CONSIDERATIONS

Exercise must be dynamic (cycling, running). Resistive or static exercise (weight lifting, handgrip) should not be used because it is associated with too small an increase in CO to get a meaningful range of pulmonary vascular pressure-flow relationships.

Exercise TTE-derived measurements of all components of PVR, including PAP, PAWP and CO should be acquired during, not after, the exercise stress, since a rapid post-exercise recovery of vascular pressure and flows normally occurs.

Body position does not matter since the same mPAP/CO slope, maximum oxygen uptake (VO₂) and maximum CO are estimated during incremental cardiopulmonary exercise testing in supine, semi-recumbent or upright positions.

The accuracy and precision of mPAP-CO slope greatly decreases using workload or VO₂ as surrogates of CO (considerable variability of CO at any given level of workload or VO₂)

From an imaging perspective, exercise TTE in the semi-recumbent position can be used safely and is the best technique

Exercise is associated with increased ventilation and pleural pressure dependent pulmonary vascular pressure swings that make the interpretation of pressure waveforms challenging.

Exercise TTE should be incremental (e.g. 20-25 Watts every 2 minutes) up to maximal workload effort in order to obtain preferably three pressure-flow coordinates.

KEY EXERCISE TTE FORMULAS

LV FUNCTION
LVEF (%)= *(LV EDV - LV ESV)LV EDV x100*

LH HEMODINAMICS
PAWP (mmHg)= 1.9 + 1.24 x average E/e'
CO= (LVOT AREA x LVOT VTI)x HR

RH HEMODINAMICS
sPAP (mmHg)= 4 x TRV² +RAP;
RAP (mmHg)= IVC diameter and collapsibility;
mPAP (mmHg)= (0.6 x sPAP +2) + RAP;
RVOT Act (msec);
mPAP/CO slope (mmHg/L/min)= (mPAP peak-mPAP rest)/ CO peak - CO rest);
PVR=TVR/VTI RVOT (cm) x 10 + 0.16

RV FUNCTION
TAPSE (mm)
RV S' TDI (cm/s)

RV-PV COUPLING
TAPSE/sPAP (mm/mmHg)

Fig. 5. Exercise Doppler echocardiography of the right heart pulmonary circulation unit: methodological insights. Key methodological requirements[8,12,26] Key formulas of exercise TTE indices.[26,42–44] AcT, acceleration time; CO, cardiac output; E, mitral inflow E velocity as measured by PW Doppler; e', early diastolic velocity of the mitral annulus as measured by TDI; EDV, end diastolic volume; EF, ejection fraction; ESV, end-systolic volume; HR, heart rate; IVC, inferior vena cava; LH, left heart; LVOT, left ventricular outflow tract; mPAP, mean pulmonary artery pressure; PAP, pulmonary artery pressure; PH, pulmonary hypertension; PVR, pulmonary vascular resistance; PW, pulsed-wave; RAP, right atrial pressure; RH, right heart; RV, right ventricle; RVOT, right ventricular outflow tract; RV-PV, right ventricular-pulmonary vascular; S', tricuspid lateral tissue Doppler imaging; sPAP, systolic pulmonary artery pressure; SV, stroke volume; TAPSE, tricuspid annular plane systolic excursion; TDI, tissue Doppler imaging; TRV, tricuspid regurgitation peak velocity; TTE, transthoracic Doppler echocardiography; VTI, velocity-time integral.

45 patients who underwent exercise RHC, E/e' 20W predicted normal PAWP during exercise (<25 mm Hg) with the cutoff value of ≤12.4, showing high specificity (83%), and an acceptable sensitivity to discriminate patients with invasively defined HFpEF from control subjects (AUC: 0.77; *P*<.01).[40]

The RIGHT-heart international NETwork meta-model

The RIGHT-NET is a large prospective clinical and exercise TTE (25W every 2 minutes on a semi-recumbent position up to maximal tolerated effort) observational multicenter study, aiming to explore

2D DOPPLER ECHO+TDI	REST	MID LEVEL EXERCISE (50-75 W; HR<110 bpm)[a]	PEAK EXERCISE
LV FUNCTION			
LV EF %	98%	—	94%
WMSI	98%	—	95%
LH HEMODINAMICS			
AVERAGE E/e'	98%	96%	VERY LOW FEASIBILITY
CO (L/min)	99.7%	96%	95%
RV FUNCTION			
TAPSE (mm)	98%	—	96%
TDI s' (cm/s)	99%	—	89%
RH HEMODINAMICS			
TRV (cm/s)	83%	—	72.3%
RVOT Act (msec)	96%	—	82%

Fig. 6. The RIGHT heart international NET-work (RIGHT-NET) protocol[41,46] CO, cardiac output; EF, ejection fraction; HR, heart rate; LH, left heart; LV, left ventricle; RV, right ventricle; RVOT, right ventricle outflow tract; TAPSE, tricuspid annular plane systolic excursion; TDI, tissue doppler imaging; TRV, tricuspid regurgitation velocity; VTI, velocity time integral; WMSI, wall motion score index; [a]Before of the E and A velocities fusion; not accessed. The numbers indicate the feasibility (%) of all indices at different level of exercise.

the physiologic versus pathologic response of the RH-PCU to exercise.[41] Key methodological considerations,[8,12,26] derived from physiologic principles, and formulas of main TTE indices[42–44] are reported in **Fig. 5**. All participating echocardiography laboratories underwent a quality control procedure with good quality reproducible results.[45] Of a note, average E/e' ratio is highly feasible at mid-level exercise (heart rate ≤110 bpm) before the E and A velocities fusion (**Fig. 6**).[41,46] So far, the RIGHT-NET study has enrolled a total of 2228 subjects including 375 healthy controls, 40 athletes, 516 patients with cardiovascular risk factors, 17 with pulmonary arterial hypertension, 872 with connective tissue diseases without overt PH, 113 with LHD, 30 with lung disease, and 265 with chronic exposure to high altitude.[27] As shown in **Fig. 2**, the lower 5th percentile of pooled normal controls and athletes were shown to have a tricuspid annular plane systolic excursion (TAPSE)/systolic pulmonary artery pressure (sPAP) of 0.7 mm/mm Hg at rest and 0.5 mm/mm Hg at peak exercise. In addition, the upper 95th percentile had an mPAP/CO slope of 3.5 mm Hg.min/L. Of note, the higher upper limits of normal of mPAP/CO slope determined by exercise TTE compared to exercise RHC may be due to the inherent lower precision of noninvasive approaches. Interestingly, an increased all-cause mortality was predicted by a TAPSE/sPAP less than .7 mm/mm Hg and mPAP–CO slope greater than 5 mm Hg.min/L.[27] Additional interesting insights are expected as this large database continues to be analyzed.

CLINICAL IMPLICATIONS

A multistep diagnostic algorithm should be considered in patients with unexplained dyspnea and/or additional symptoms/signs raising suspicion of PH (**Fig. 7**).[2] In this regard, resting TTE is essential in determining the probability of PH (high, intermediate, and low), based on an abnormal TRV and the presence of other echocardiographic signs suggestive of PH. Further testing should be considered according to the clinical context (see **Fig. 7**).[2] In the case of patients with unexplained dyspnea and intermediate echocardiographic probability of PH, exercise TTE may be particularly useful. If exercise TRV is less than 3.4 m/s and/or mPAP/CO slope less than 3.5 mm Hg/L/min, exercise PH could be ruled out with reasonable certainty. Furthermore, exercise average E/e' less than 15 may exclude LV diastolic dysfunction as cause of exercise increase of

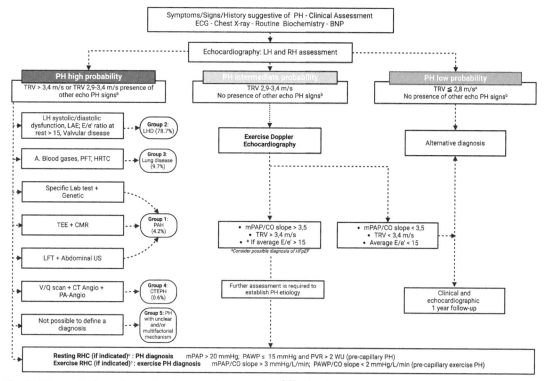

Fig. 7. Diagnostic flow-chart of pulmonary hypertension.[2,20] BNP, brain natriuretic peptide; CMR, cardiac magnetic resonance; CO, cardiac output; CT, computed tomography; CTEPH, chronic thrombo-embolic pulmonary hypertension; ECG, electrocardiogram; echo, echocardiography; HRTC, high resolution computed tomography; LAE, left atrial enlargement; LFT, liver functional test; LH, left heart; LHD, left heart disease; mPAP, mean pulmonary artery pressure; PA, pulmonary artery; PAH, pulmonary arterial hypertension; PAWP, pulmonary artery wedge pressure; PFT, pulmonary function test; PH, pulmonary hypertension; PVR, pulmonary vascular resistance; RH, right heart; RHC, right heart catheterization; TEE, transesophageal echocardiography; TRV, tricuspid regurgitation velocity; US, ultrasound; WU, Wood units. [a]Or unmeasurable; [b]Other echocardiographic signs from at least 2 categories (A/B/C) must be present to alter the level of echocardiographic probability of PH: The ventricle (A) = RV/LV basal diameter/area ratio greater than 1.0; Flattening of the interventricular septum (LV eccentricity index >1.1 in systole and/or diastole, TAPSE/sPAP ratio < 0.55 mm/mm Hg; Pulmonary artery (B) = RVOT AT less than 105 ms and/or mid-systolic notching; early diastolic pulmonary regurgitation velocity greater than 2.2 m/s; PA diameter greater than 25 mm. Inferior vena cava and RA (C) = IVC diameter greater than 21 mm with decreased inspiratory collapse (<50% with a sniff or <20% with quiet inspiration; RA area (end-systole) greater than 18 cm². [c]RHC should be performed if useful information/a therapeutic consequence is anticipated. It is particularly indicated in a small subset of patients with suspected pulmonary arterial hypertension (group 1) and chronic thromboembolic pulmonary hypertension, before starting specific therapies and/or pulmonary endarterectomy (PEA) surgery. In patients with PH associated to LHD, the RHC is only indicated in the following cases: (a) suspected combined post-capillary and pre-capillary PH with a severe pre-capillary component, if it aids management decisions; (b) severe tricuspid regurgitation with or without LHD prior to surgical or interventional valve repair; (c) advanced HF and evaluation for heart transplantation.[2]

pulmonary pressure (see **Fig. 7**).[2] In this regard, the Heart Failure Association Pretest assessment, Echocardiography & natriuretic peptide, Functional testing, Final etiology (HFA-PEFF) diagnostic algorithm recommends that, in patient with exertional dyspnea, LV diastolic dysfunction may be unmasked during exercise if average E/e' ratio is greater than 15, with or without TRV greater than 3.4 m/sec.[20,39] It should be highlighted that exercise RHC should be undertaken in a high-specialized center if a therapeutic decision is dependent on the results.[2]

SUMMARY AND FUTURE DIRECTIONS

Pulmonary vascular pressures are flow-dependent with invasively determined upper limits of normal for mPAP and PAWP as a function of CO relationships of 3 mm Hg/L/min and 2 mm Hg/L/min, respectively. Although exercise RHC remains the gold standard, exercise TTE is the most widely available and sustainable non-invasive test. Further studies are needed to develop a multiparametric model, including exercise TTE-derived pressure-flow slopes that may more accurately allow differentiation of a normal versus abnormal RH-PCU response to exercise.

CLINICS CARE POINTS

- Exercise pulmonary hypertension has been invasively defined as mean pulmonary artery pressure/cardiac output slope greater than 3 mm Hg/L/min.

- Although exercise right-heart catheterization remains the gold standard, exercise pulmonary hypertension could be rule out with reasonable certainty if exercise Doppler echocardiographic-derived mean pulmonary artery pressure/cardiac output slope is less than 3.5 mm Hg/L min and tricuspid regurgitation velocity is less than 3.4 m/s.

- Exercise average E/e′ greater than 15 may detect left ventricular diastolic dysfunction as cause of exercise increase of pulmonary pressure.

DISCLOSURES

The authors have nothing to disclose.

REFERENCES

1. Picano E, Pierard L, Peteiro J, et al. The clinical use of stress echocardiography in chronic coronary syndromes and beyond coronary artery disease: a clinical consensus statement from the European Association of Cardiovascular Imaging of the ESC. Eur Heart J Cardiovasc Imaging 2024;25(2):e65–90.
2. Humbert M, Kovacs G, Hoeper MM, et al. 2022 ESC/ERS Guidelines for the diagnosis and treatment of pulmonary hypertension. Eur Heart J 2022;43:3618–31.
3. Bossone E, Naeije R. Exercise-induced pulmonary hypertension. Heart Fail Clin 2012;8:485–95.
4. Reeves JT, Dempsey JA, Grover RF. Pulmonary circulation during exercise. In: Weir EK, Reeves JT, editors. Pulmonary vascular physiology and physiopathology. New York: Marcel Dekker; 1989. p. 107–33. chap 4.
5. Argiento P, Vanderpool RR, Mulè M, et al. Exercise stress echocardiography of the pulmonary circulation: limits of normal and sex differences. Chest 2012;142:1158–65.
6. Zeder K, Banfi C, Steinrisser-Allex G, et al. Diagnostic, prognostic and differential-diagnostic relevance of pulmonary haemodynamic parameters during exercise: a systematic review. Eur Respir J 2022;60:2103181.
7. Lewis GD, Bossone E, Naeije R, et al. Pulmonary vascular hemodynamic response to exercise in cardiopulmonary diseases. Circulation 2013;128:1470–9.
8. Naeije R, Saggar R, Badesch D, et al. Exercise-Induced Pulmonary Hypertension: Translating Pathophysiological Concepts Into Clinical Practice. Chest 2018;154:10–5.
9. Vonk-Noordegraaf A, Haddad F, Chin KM, et al. Right heart adaptation to pulmonary arterial hypertension: physiology and pathobiology. J Am Coll Cardiol 2013;62:D22–33.
10. Bossone E, Rubenfire M, Bach DS, et al. Range of tricuspid regurgitation velocity at rest and during exercise in normal adult men: implications for the diagnosis of pulmonary hypertension. J Am Coll Cardiol 1999;33:1662–6.
11. West JB. Vulnerability of pulmonary capillaries during exercise. Exerc Sport Sci Rev 2004;32:24–30.
12. Kovacs G, Herve P, Barbera JA, et al. An official European Respiratory Society statement: pulmonary haemodynamics during exercise. Eur Respir J 2017;50:1700578.
13. Forton K, Motoji Y, Deboeck G, et al. Effects of body position on exercise capacity and pulmonary vascular pressure-flow relationships. J Appl Physiol 2016;121:1145–50.
14. Berry NC, Manyoo A, Oldham WM, et al. Protocol for exercise hemodynamic assessment: performing an invasive cardiopulmonary exercise test in clinical practice. Pulm Circ 2015;5:610–8.
15. Wright SP, Esfandiari S, Gray T, et al. The pulmonary artery wedge pressure response to sustained exercise is time-variant in healthy adults. Heart 2016;102:438–43.
16. Esfandiari S, Wright SP, Goodman JM, et al. Pulmonary artery wedge pressure relative to exercise work rate in older men and women. Med Sci Sports Exerc 2017;49:1297–304.
17. Wolsk E, Bakkestrøm R, Thomsen JH, et al. The influence of age on hemodynamic parameters during rest and exercise in healthy individuals. JACC Heart Fail 2017;5:337–46.
18. Andersen MJ, Wolsk E, Bakkestrøm R, et al. Hemodynamic response to rapid saline infusion compared with exercise in healthy participants aged 20–80 years. J Card Fail 2019;25:902–10.
19. Borlaug BA, Nishimura RA, Sorajja P, et al. Exercise hemodynamics enhance diagnosis of early heart failure with preserved ejection fraction. Circ Heart Fail 2010;3:588–95.
20. Pieske B, Tschope C, de Boer RA, et al. How to diagnose heart failure with preserved ejection fraction: the HFA-PEFF diagnostic algorithm:a consensus recommendation from the Heart Failure Association (HFA), of the European Society of Cardiology (ESC). Eur Heart J 2019;40:3297–317.

21. Baratto C, Caravita S, Soranna D, et al. Exercise haemodynamics in heart failure with preserved ejection fraction: a systematic review and meta-analysis. ESC Heart Fail 2022;9:3079–91.

22. Ehrsam RE, Perruchoud A, Oberholzer M, et al. Influence of age on pulmonary haemodynamics at rest and during supine exercise. Clin Sci (Lond) 1983;65:653–60.

23. Eisman AS, Shah RV, Dhakal BP, et al. Pulmonary capillary wedge pressure patterns during exercise predict exercise capacity and incident heart failure. Circ Heart Fail 2018;11:e004750.

24. Picano E. Economic, ethical, and environmental sustainability of cardiac imaging. Eur Heart J 2023;44:4748–51.

25. Lancellotti P, Pellikka PA, Budts W, et al. The Clinical Use of Stress Echocardiography in Non-Ischaemic Heart Disease: Recommendations from the European Association of Cardiovascular Imaging and the American Society of Echocardiography. J Am Soc Echocardiogr 2017;30:101–38.

26. Rudski LG, Gargani L, Armstrong WF, et al. Stressing the cardiopulmonary vascular system: the role of echocardiography. JASE 2018;31:527–50.

27. Gargani L, Pugliese NR, De Biase N, et al. RIGHT Heart International NETwork (RIGHT-NET) Investigators. Exercise Stress Echocardiography of the Right Ventricle and Pulmonary Circulation. J Am Coll Cardiol 2023;82:1973–85.

28. Kovacs G, Maier R, Aberer E, et al. Assessment of pulmonary arterial pressure during exercise in collagen vascular disease: echocardiography vs right-sided heart catheterization. Chest 2010;138:270–8.

29. Claessen G, La Gerche A, Voigt JU, et al. Accuracy of echocardiography to evaluate pulmonary vascular and RV function during exercise. JACC Cardiovasc Imaging 2016;9:532–43.

30. van Riel AC, Opotowsky AR, Santos M, et al. Accuracy of echocardiography to estimate pulmonary artery pressures with exercise: a simultaneous invasive-noninvasive comparison. Circ Cardiovasc Imaging 2017;10:e005711.

31. Grünig E, Weissmann S, Ehlken N, et al. Stress Doppler echocardiography in relatives of patients with idiopathic and familial pulmonary arterial hypertension: results of a multicenter European analysis of pulmonary artery pressure response to exercise and hypoxia. Circulation 2009;119:1747–57.

32. Mahjoub H, Levy F, Cassol M, et al. Effects of age on pulmonary artery systolic pressure at rest and during exercise in normal adults. Eur J Echocardiogr 2009;10:635–40.

33. D'Alto M, Ghio S, D'Andrea A, et al. Inappropriate exercise-induced increase in pulmonary artery pressure in patients with systemic sclerosis. Heart 2011;97:112–7.

34. Chia EM, Lau EM, Xuan W, et al. Exercise testing can unmask right ventricular dysfunction in systemic sclerosis patients with normal resting pulmonary artery pressure. Int J Cardiol 2016;204:179–86.

35. D'Alto M, Pavelescu A, Argiento P, et al. Echocardiographic assessment of right ventricular contractile reserve in healthy subjects. Echocardiography 2017;34:61–8.

36. D'Andrea A, Stanziola AA, Saggar R, et al. Right ventricular functional reserve in early-stage idiopathic pulmonary fibrosis: an exercise two-dimensional speckle tracking doppler echocardiography study. Chest 2019;155:297–306.

37. Wierzbowska-Drabik K, Kasprzak JD, D Alto M, et al. Reduced pulmonary vascular reserve during stress echocardiography in confirmed pulmonary hypertension and patients at risk of overt pulmonary hypertension. Int J Cardiovasc Imag 2020;36:1831–43.

38. Vriz O, Palatini P, Rudski L, et al. Right Heart Pulmonary Circulation Unit Response to Exercise in Patients with Controlled Systemic Arterial Hypertension: Insights from the RIGHT Heart International NETwork (RIGHT-NET). J Clin Med 2022;11:451.

39. Obokata M, Olson TP, Reddy YNV, et al. Haemodynamics, dyspnoea, and pulmonary reserve in heart failure with preserved ejection fraction. Eur Heart J 2018;39:2810–21.

40. Harada T, Obokata M, Kagami K, et al. Utility of E/e' ratio during low-level exercise to diagnose heart failure with preserved ejection fraction. JACC Cardiovasc Imaging 2022. S1936-878X(22)00666-0.

41. Ferrara F, Gargani L, Armstrong WF, et al. The Right Heart International Network (RIGHT-NET): Rationale, Objectives, Methodology, and Clinical Implications. Heart Fail Clin 2018;14:443–65.

42. Rudski LG, Lai WW, Afilalo J, et al. Guidelines for the echocardiographic assessment of the right heart in adults: a report from the American Society of Echocardiography endorsed by the European Association of Echocardiography, a registered branch of the European Society of Cardiology, and the Canadian Society of Echocardiography. J Am Soc Echocardiogr 2010;23:685–713.

43. Lang RM, Badano LP, Mor-Avi V, et al. Recommendations for cardiac chamber quantification by echocardiography in adults: an update from the American Society of Echocardiography and the European Association of Cardiovascular Imaging. J Am Soc Echocardiogr 2015;28:1–39.e14.

44. Nagueh SF, Smiseth OA, Appleton CP, et al. Recommendations for the evaluation of left ventricular diastolic function by echocardiography: an update from the american society of echocardiography and the european association of cardiovascular imaging. J Am Soc Echocardiogr 2016;29:277–314.

45. Ferrara F, Gargani L, Contaldi C, et al. A multicentric quality-control study of exercise Doppler echocardiography of the right heart and the pulmonary circulation. The RIGHT Heart International NETwork (RIGHT-NET). Cardiovasc Ultrasound 2021;19:9.

46. Ferrara F, Gargani L, Naeije R, et al. Feasibility of semi-recumbent bicycle exercise Doppler echocardiography for the evaluation of the right heart and pulmonary circulation unit in different clinical conditions: the RIGHT heart international NETwork (RIGHT-NET). Int J Cardiovasc Imag 2021;37(7):2151–67.

Exercise Testing in Elite Athletes

Eric Rudofker, MD[a], Natalie Van Ochten, MD[b], Justin Edward, MD[a,c], Hugh Parker, MD[a], Kyla Wulff, BSN, RN[d], Emmett Suckow, BS[a], Lindsey Forbes, MD[e], William K. Cornwell III, MD, MSCS[a,d,*]

KEYWORDS

- Exercise testing • Athletes • Fitness • Cardiovascular disease

KEY POINTS

- A lifelong commitment to exercise leads to unique cardiovascular adaptations, including alterations in structure and function, commonly referred to as the "athletic heart."
- Athletes may require exercise testing for a variety of reasons including evaluation of exertional symptoms, identifying ventilatory threshold and maximal oxygen uptake, and/or to establish training zones to improve fitness and performance during competition.
- Cardiopulmonary exercise testing should be tailored appropriately to athletes, since their physiologic response to exercise is unique when compared to other populations (eg, cardiovascular and/or pulmonary vascular disease) who are referred for testing.

INTRODUCTION

Exercise testing with heart rate (HR) and blood pressure monitoring was first described in 1929; electrocardiography monitoring was subsequently added and became the standard test in the evaluation of coronary disease in the 1950s.[1–3] Since those early applications, the utility of exercise testing has broadened to a number of disease states spanning the spectrum of health and disease, including endurance athletes, healthy control populations, individuals with risk factors for cardiovascular disease (CVD), pulmonary and pulmonary vascular disease,[4] ambulatory and advanced heart failure (HF), as well as cardiomyopathies (eg, hypertrophic cardiomyopathy) and patients with conduction abnormalities (eg, Wolff–Parkinson–White syndrome, Long QT syndrome).[5] Testing in

these populations provides prognostic information and informs management strategies specific to the patient's risk profile and disease status.[6–8]

Athletes represent a unique population for which cardiopulmonary exercise testing (CPET) may be useful for a variety of reasons, such as evaluation of symptoms during exercise; distinguishing the athletic heart from an acquired cardiomyopathy; formulation of exercise prescriptions and training zones; and monitoring exercise capacity overtime. The term "athlete" does not have a standard definition, and while the exact definition is debated,[9,10] generally, the term is applied to individuals engaging in any number of sporting disciplines based on the level of dynamic and static load[11,12] with varying levels of duration/intensity of their respective sport, including elite, recreationally active, and even weekend warriors.[13] In

[a] Department of Medicine-Cardiology, University of Colorado Anschutz Medical Campus, 12631 East 17th Avenue, Aurora 80045, USA; [b] Department of Medicine, University of Colorado Anschutz Medical Campus, 12631 East 17th Avenue, Aurora 80045, USA; [c] Department of Cardiology, Kaiser Permanente, 2045 Franklin Street, # 200, Denver, CO 80205, USA; [d] Clinical Translational Research Center, University of Colorado Anschutz Medical Campus, 12401 East 17th Avenue Leprino Building, Aurora, CO, USA; [e] Division of Pulmonary and Critical Care Medicine, Department of Medicine, University of Colorado Anschutz Medical Campus, 12631 East 17th Avenue, Aurora 80045, USA
* Corresponding author.
E-mail address: William.Cornwell@cuanschutz.edu

Heart Failure Clin 21 (2025) 15–25
https://doi.org/10.1016/j.hfc.2024.05.001

this review, the authors discuss physiologic adaptations to exercise, variations in phenotype of the athletic heart, and considerations for CPET in this unique population.

CARDIOVASCULAR RESPONSE TO EXERCISE

The ability to engage in, and sustain physical work, requires mobilization of atmospheric oxygen into the exercising muscle for generation of adenosine triphosphate (ATP) to support the metabolic demands of the body. The "oxygen cascade" describes the multiple components of this system and series of steps by which this process occurs. Essential features of the cascade include the following[14–16]:

1. Atmospheric partial pressure of oxygen
2. Interface between the environment and body at the level of the lung and ventilation
3. Diffusion of oxygen from the alveoli into pulmonary capillaries into the blood
4. Binding of oxygen to hemoglobin (Hgb)
5. Delivery of oxygen to the body by the cardiovascular system
6. Diffusion of oxygen into the skeletal muscle through skeletal muscle capillaries
7. Oxidative phosphorylation within mitochondria to generate ATP

The Fick equation describes the relationship between oxygen uptake (VO_2), cardiac output (Qc), Hgb, and oxygen uptake in the periphery (AVO_{2diff}):

$$VO_2 = Qc \times Hgb \times AVO_{2diff}$$

The relationship between VO_2 and Qc is inviolate, and regardless of age and gender, for every 1 L/min increase in VO_2 during exercise, Qc increases by 5–6 L/min.[17–19] This relationship between VO_2 and Qc is maintained across the spectrum of health and CVD, except potentially in cases of advanced HF and impending decompensation.[16] Thus, the measure of maximal exercise capacity (VO_{2max}) can be viewed as a surrogate measure of maximal Qc during exercise.

In terms of exercise performance, "economy" refers to the relationship between VO_2 and work rate and varies according to the type of exercise. Economy generally describes energy expenditure necessary for a given exercise intensity. An individual with poor economy requires a large amount of VO_2 to complete any level of work, while a trained athlete with good economy requires less VO_2 for the same level of work (**Fig. 1**).[20] Different exercise types also vary in energy expenditure for work required. For example, walking and cycling are very economical.[16] However, running is less efficient, meaning that a greater VO_2 is required for

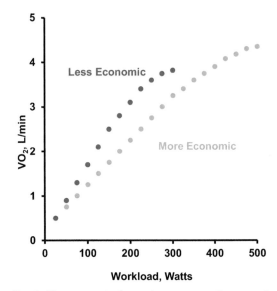

Fig. 1. The concept of exercise economy. Economy is described by the relationship between VO_2 and workload. In this model, an athlete with good economy requires less VO_2 for any level of work compared to a nonathletic individual, who requires greater VO_2 for the same level of work.

useful work, and among swimmers, as little as 10% of energy production is used for actual work.[21] As work intensity increases and approaches maximal effort, VO_2 plateaus, such that further increases in work rate do not translate to any additional increase in VO_2. This value represents the maximum rate of oxygen uptake, or VO_{2max}.

Maximal Steady State and Submaximal Exercise

As exercise intensity increases, there exists a threshold level beyond which exercise cannot be sustained for prolonged periods of time. This threshold may be of particular relevance to athletes as it relates to training zones and determining performance levels for competition. Several terms have been used to describe this cutoff point, including "ventilatory threshold" (VT), "anaerobic threshold" (AT), and "lactate threshold" or onset of blood lactate accumulation (OBLA). All of these terms have gained popularity and generally describe a similar concept related to a threshold of exercise intensity above which it is not possible to sustain exercise. While an in-depth analysis of these terms and the relevant physiology is beyond the scope of this review, there are a few key points that are important to emphasize in the context of exercise physiology in the athlete.

First, minute ventilation (V_E), readily measured during CPET, provides critical insight into exercise intensity and the physiologic adaptations required to sustain work. As work intensity increases, VT is identified as the point in time when the rate of increase in V_E exceeds the rate of increase in VO_2 (**Fig. 2**).[16] VT is often more specifically broken down into VT1 and VT2. VT1 represents the workload at which lactate begins to rise in the blood, as well as the increase in V_E required to meet the increased demand of oxygen delivery and CO_2 export. VT1 is identified as the point in time when the ventilatory equivalent of oxygen (V_E/VO_2) reaches a nadir and then increases without an increase in the ventilatory equivalent of carbon dioxide (V_E/VCO_2). VT1 may also be determined by identifying an increase in the slope of VCO_2 compared to VO_2 (ie, the V-slope method). The increase in VCO_2 results from lactate buffering.[22,23] VT2 is identified by the point where V_E/VCO_2 nadirs and then begins to increase. VT2 represents the period of time when lactate rapidly rises, resulting in hyperventilation.[22–24] This point signifies the workload at, and above which, there is a disproportionate rise in V_E relative to continued increases in workload and VO_2. The increase in V_E is driven by the heightened CO_2 production resulting from hydrogen ion buildup during exercise.[24]

The second point is in regard to lactate metabolism. Lactate exists almost completely dissociated into lactate and hydrogen ion (H+) due to a low pK. H^+ ions are buffered by bicarbonate (HCO_3^-), generating carbonic acid (H_2CO_3) and CO_2 according to the following reaction[25]:

$$H^+ + HCO_3^- \leftrightarrows H_2CO_3 \leftrightarrows CO_2 + H_2O$$

During very low-intensity exercise, lactate—a product of glycolytic metabolism—remains low at/near resting levels. At slightly higher levels of intensity—but still well below maximal steady state, lactate production increases in response to

pyruvate production (during accelerated glycolysis) but levels remain low since production is offset by clearance. With workloads above VT2, lactate production exceeds the buffering capacity of bicarbonate. This point is referred to as the lactate threshold, or OBLA,[16] and can be identified during an incremental exercise test by measuring blood lactate levels. At this point, peripheral chemoreceptors (in response to the metabolic acidosis) promote hyperventilation, visible by a rapid/exponential increase in V_E. For this reason, VT2 is also referred to as the respiratory compensation point and represents the maximum steady state—that is, the work intensity that can be sustained for prolonged periods of time.[20]

Finally, there is no "threshold" of exercise—or point in time, where the body shifts completely from aerobic to anaerobic metabolism, meaning that there is no point in time where energy production shifts suddenly from oxidative phosphorylation to glycolysis. Rather, the exponential increase in blood lactate concentration (ie, the lactate threshold) occurs due to increased rate of pyruvate production and glycolytic flux in response to increases in work intensity. However, it does not indicate an absence of aerobic metabolism at high workloads. While the concept of an "anaerobic threshold" may sound convenient to use in the clinical realm, physiologically, there is no threshold characterized by a complete transition to anaerobic metabolism to meet metabolic demand.[16]

HR is probably the easiest physiologic variable that can be followed during an incremental exercise test. HR increases linearly with VO_2 uptake and rises in response to multiple factors. With onset of exercise, HR increases due to both sympathetic activation and parasympathetic withdrawal. The rate of increase in HR varies according to an individual's level of fitness. For example, sedentary and/or

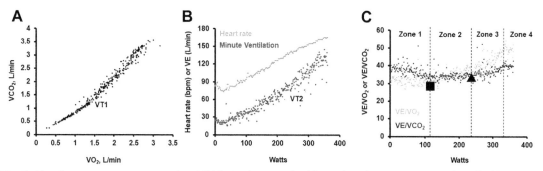

Fig. 2. Ventilatory response to exercise. (*A*) The V-slope method is used to determine VT1 and marked by an increase in VCO_2 in relation to VO_2 that results from an increase in lactate accumulation. (*B*) VT2 may be visualized by a deflection point in the HR as it begins to level off (the Conconi HR) and a marked increase in ventilation due to rapid accumulation of lactate. (*C*) Based on the ventilatory response to exercise, training zones may be developed in relation to VT1 (square) and VT2 (triangle). Here, VT1 is signified by the nadir in V_E/VO_2 and VT2 is signified by the nadir in V_E/VCO_2. See text for further details.

deconditioned patients experience a rapid rise in HR with onset of exercise, whereas among trained individuals, the increase in HR in response to exercise is more gradual. As exercise intensity increases, the rate of rise of HR levels off, particularly as the maximal exercise capacity is approached. This deflection point in HR, also referred to as the Conconi HR, coincides with the accumulation of blood lactate and, in this regard, may serve as an indirect method of determining the maximum steady state in athletes.[26]

The Athletic Heart: Cardiovascular Remodeling in Response to Exercise Training

Cardiac size and structure may vary among athletes depending on the type, intensity and duration of exercise, and fitness as determined by VO_{2max}.[27,28] Morganroth and colleagues were the first to characterize variations in cardiac structure and function among athletes engaging in different types of exercise.[29] Using echocardiography, they found that left ventricle (LV) end-diastolic volume (LVEDV) and mass were increased among athletes engaging in dynamic types of exercise, whereas wall thickness and mass were increased among athletes participating in static types of exercise (but LVEDV was normal).[29] Differences in cardiac structure according to sport type have been attributed to variations in cardiac loading conditions placed upon the heart (**Fig. 3**). Dynamic exercises promote eccentric hypertrophy with increased LVEDV resulting from repetitive exposure to increased Qc and a volume load on the heart.[11] Static exercises promote concentric hypertrophy with increased wall thickness resulting from repetitive exposure to increased total peripheral resistance and a pressure load on the heart.[11,29] That said, the majority of sport types have significant overlap in their components of dynamic and static exercise, and consequently, any individual's remodeling pattern will vary accordingly, not fitting neatly into one extreme or the other.[28,30–33]

Multiple studies evaluating cardiac structure and function have followed Morganroth's initial report.[29,31,33] In a systematic review and meta-analysis, Fagard found that compared to controls, LV mass was 64% greater among cyclists, 48% greater among runners, and 25% greater in strength-trained athletes.[31] In another meta-analysis, Pluim and colleagues[33] stratified athletes (N = 1451) into one of 3 groups based on exercise type: purely dynamic, purely static, or combined, and compared these groups to nonathletic controls. In this analysis, athletes engaged in combined dynamic/static had the largest cardiac mass (288 g) compared to athletes engaged in

static exercise (267 g) and endurance-trained athletes (249 g) and nonathletic controls (174 g).[33]

Right ventricular (RV) enlargement also occurs in response to endurance exercise, supporting the concept of "balanced dilatation."[28,34–36] Multiple studies of endurance athletes have demonstrated that the RV is generally enlarged when compared to nonathletic controls.[35,37–39] In one analysis using cardiac MRI, compared to controls, endurance athletes had greater RV mass (77±10 vs 56±8 g) and RV end-diastolic volume (160±26 vs 128±10 mL).[40] Similar findings have been reported among other athletes participating in exercises such as orienteering, cross-country skiing, or middle-distance running.[41] Static exercise types, however, do not appear to lead to hypertrophy of the RV.[36,42] In an analysis of collegiate athletes engaging in rowing (N = 40) versus American football (N = 40), echocardiogram prior to and following 3 months of exercise training, demonstrated that rowers experienced an increase in RV end-diastolic area (pre vs post: 1460±220 vs 1650±200 mm/m^2), while football players had no change in RV size.[42]

The RV, a thin-walled and highly compliant chamber, has substantial contractile reserve and significantly augments contractility during exercise.[43,44] In an invasive CPET of healthy individuals, conductance catheters inserted into the RV demonstrated an approximate 4 fold increase in metrics of contractility during exercise, as well as myocardial energy production (**Fig. 4**).[43] However, prolonged exercise—for example, during endurance races (eg, marathons, triathlons)—disproportionately stresses the RV compared to the LV due to sustained increases in pulmonary arterial pressures—and hence, RV afterload.[45–50] In a study of endurance athletes (N = 40) competing in events 3 to 11 hours duration, LV volumes and systolic function remained stable following completion of the event, but RV volumes increased and metrics of RV systolic function (ejection fraction, tricuspid annular plane systolic excursion) declined when compared to baseline, prerace values.[46] Among these athletes, the reduction in RV systolic function was dose dependent, such that athletes completing races of 11 hours had greater declines in RV systolic function compared to athletes completing shorter events, such as a marathon (3 hours) or triathlon (5.5 hours).[46] Invasive CPET simulating endurance competition has elegantly demonstrated acquired RV dysfunction based on real-time RV pressure–volume analysis.[50] In a meta-analysis of studies (N = 14) evaluating LV and RV function following at least 90 minutes of exercise, LV function remained stable, but RV function declined following completion of the event, with reductions in RV

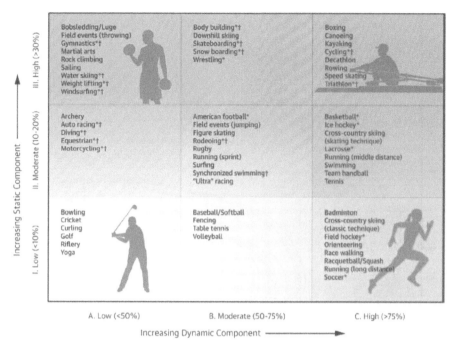

Fig. 3. The classification of different sports/exercises is based on the relative contribution of static versus dynamic exercise intensity. The dynamic component of exercise refers to the estimated percentage of maximal oxygen uptake (VO_{2max}) achieved during exercise and results in an increased cardiac output. The static component of exercise is related to the percentage of maximal voluntary contraction achieved during effort and results in an increased blood pressure load and total peripheral resistance. * Indicates, Danger of bodily collision. Cross indicates, Increased risk if syncope occurs. (*Reprinted from* Levine et al[11] with permission.)

fractional area by 5.78% (4.46%–7.09%), RV ejection fraction by 7.05% (1.2%–12.3%), and tricuspid annular plane systolic excursion by 4.77 mm (1.24–8.3 mm).[49] These reductions in RV systolic function appear to be reversible, with available data indicating return to normal function about a week after recovery.[46,48]

Ventricular Function in the Athletic Heart

A lifelong commitment to exercise favorably influences ventricular lusitropy. In a cross-sectional analysis, healthy seniors (N = 102) approximately 67 to 70 years of age were stratified into 1 of 4 groups according to lifelong patterns of exercise training: "sedentary" (<2 sessions/week); "casual" (2–3 sessions per week); "committed" (4–5 sessions per week); or "competitive" Masters athletes (6–7 sessions per week).[51] Participants completed invasive hemodynamic and echocardiographic assessment of LV structure and function. Overall, LV distensibility was greater in committed and competitive exercisers than sedentary individuals (**Fig. 5**).[51] Furthermore, LV stiffness constants were increased among sedentary individuals when compared to competitive Masters athletes, and LV compliance was greater among competitive

Masters athletes and committed exercisers than sedentary or casual exercisers.[51] These very elegant data demonstrate the beneficial effects of a lifelong commitment to exercise of at least 4 to 5 times per week—namely a preservation of ventricular compliance in the elderly years; and also, the consequences of sedentary aging—specifically, an increase in LV stiffness and reduction in distensibility and compliance.[51] Similar findings were observed in another analysis of middle aged (53±5 years) previously sedentary healthy individuals (N = 53) who were randomized to 2 years of exercise versus control with yoga.[52] Exercise was primarily a combination of high-intensity interval training and moderate continuous exercise with a combination of running, cycling, ellipticals, and/or swimming.[52] Compared to the control group, exercisers experienced reductions in LV stiffness as evidenced by a down/rightward shift in the diastolic limb of an LV pressure–volume curve. In this same analysis, exercise also increased LVEDV.[52]

Atrial Remodeling and Risk of Atrial Fibrillation

In addition to ventricular remodeling with exercise, the left atrium (LA) may also undergo structural

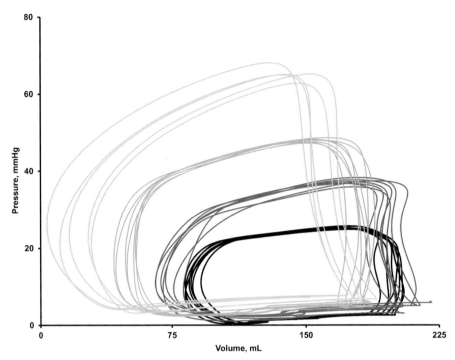

Fig. 4. Right ventricular pressure–volume analysis during exercise. Real-time right ventricular pressure–volume analysis during invasive CPET from a healthy 26 year old man during upright cycle ergometry. Black represents rest; red and blue represent 2 levels of submaximal exercise below VT, and gold represents peak effort. As workload increases, right ventricular stroke volume increases as evidenced by a progressive increase in width of the pressure–volume loop. (Cornwell, W.K. et al., (2020), New insights into resting and exertional right ventricular performance in the healthy heart through real-time pressure-volume analysis. J Physiol, 598: 2575-2587.)

remodeling in response to exercise, increasing the risk of atrial fibrillation (AF) in athletes.[12] In a large analysis 1,777 competitive athletes competing in an array of sports (38 different events), 347 (20%) had evidence of LA enlargement.[53] Athletes with enlarged LA were predominantly men and with larger body surface area, and while these athletes competed in a variety of 28 different sports,

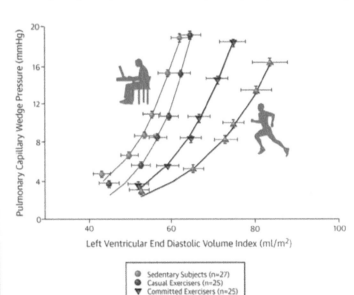

Fig. 5. Left ventricular compliance according to lifelong "dose" of exercise. Left ventricular end-diastolic pressure–volume relationship, reconstructed from invasive hemodynamic assessment and echocardiogram demonstrating increased compliance among healthy seniors who were competitive exercisers (exercising 6–7 sessions/week throughout adult life) and committed exercisers (exercising 4–5 sessions/week throughout adult life) compared to casual exercisers (exercising 2–3 sessions/week throughout adult life) and sedentary individuals. (*Reprinted from* Bhella et al[51] with permission.)

most engaged in rowing/canoeing (18%), cycling (10%), ice hockey (10%), rugby (7%), and soccer (7%).[53]

In the population at large, there is a U-shaped relationship between exercise and risk of AF.[54–60] While routine physical activity reduces the risk of incident AF, among committed exercisers, the risk increases and approximates the risk observed in the general population. Multiple factors may contribute to AF in athletes, including atrial dilatation, fibrosis, and myocardial inflammation that leads to development of an atrial myopathy.[61,62] LA dilatation, a well-recognized factor predisposing to AF, is a hallmark of the athletic heart.[28,63] Myocardial inflammation occurs in a dose-dependent manner with exercise duration and intensity.[64,65]

Concern over the increased risk of AF among competitive athletes has led to investigations into whether the risk of stroke is also increased in athletes with AF.[12] In one very large analysis, the rates of AF and stroke were compared between Swedish skiers (N = 208,654) completing a cross-country skiing event 30–90 km and nonathletic controls (N = 527,488).[66] The authors reported several important findings into the complex relationship among exercise, AF, and stroke risk. First, athletes with AF had a higher incidence of stroke than athletes/controls without AF (men: hazard ratio [HR] 2.28; 95% confidence interval [CI] 1.93 to 2.70; women HR 3.51, 95% CI 2.17 to 5.68). Second, among all individuals (athletes plus controls) with AF, athletes with AF had a lower incidence of stroke (HR 0.73, 95% CI 0.50–0.91) as well as a lower mortality than controls with AF (HR 0.57, 95% CI 0.49–0.65).[66] This observation supports the concept that despite the fact that a lifelong commitment to exercise is associated with an increased risk of AF, exercise reduces the risk and severity of comorbidities that otherwise contribute to the increased risk of adverse outcomes (eg, mortality, vascular events) in the nonathletic population.[67]

CONSIDERATIONS FOR EXERCISE TESTING IN ATHLETES

While indications for stress testing and CPET in the general population are well described,[7] there are several unique considerations for stress testing athletes, such as assessments of overall fitness, establishing training zones, evaluating exertional symptoms (angina, dyspnea, palpitations, syncope), and establishing risk of sudden cardiac death.[68] By virtue of their training history, athletes possess higher levels of performance and also are uniquely trained in a variety of sporting disciplines. As such, protocols and implementation strategies

for conducting stress tests in this unique population are different than the general population, and as such, additional measures are warranted to ensure that studies are appropriately executed. The protocol selected should adequately reproduce the physiologic demands and conditions experienced during training and competition. The Bruce protocol, frequently implemented for standard stress testing, likely is not the most appropriate exercise protocol to use.[69] Other protocols, such as the Astrand or Costill/Fox protocols, may be more appropriate for athletes,[68,69] and it may be necessary to further customize protocols according to an individual athlete's training regimen and sport type.

Determining Maximal Effort on a Cardiopulmonary Exercise Testing

The traditional criterion utilized for determining maximal effort on a stress test is an arbitrary cutoff of 85% maximum predicted HR achieved.[70] However, an exercise test should not be stopped by the test proctor simply because this arbitrary threshold has been achieved, as it does not necessarily represent a true effort since test subjects can frequently continue exercising at higher workloads.[68,70] Rather, HR is only one of several factors that should be taken into consideration. A peak/maximal effort on stress testing is suggested by the following[7,16,68,71]:

- Plateau of VO_2 despite increasing workloads
- Respiratory exchange ratio (ratio of VCO_2 and VO_2) exceeding 1.10
- Lactate concentration (when measured) of 8 mmol/L or greater
- Rate of perceived exertion of 18 or greater on the Borg Category scale or 8 or greater on the Borg Category–Ratio Scale

These factors should all be considered when CPET is performed for athletes, particularly when the goal of the test is to identify mechanisms of exertional symptoms. That said, a plateau/leveling of the VO_2 and workload relationship is the gold-standard metric for determining maximal effort. Other factors may be limited by interindividual variability.[71]

Cardiopulmonary Exercise Testing Findings Unique to Athletes

Several aspects of CPET are unique to athletes as a result of cardiorespiratory and exercise physiology in well-trained individuals. The first aspect is in regard to VT. In the general population, VT occurs around 55% to 65% of VO_{2max}; however, in trained athletes, VT may occur at a much greater percentage of VO_{2max}.[68] Athletes reporting symptoms when returning to competition after detraining and with evidence of a reduced VT and VO_{2max} may be suffering from deconditioning (in the absence of any other objective findings). The second point is in regard to breathing reserve. V_E during CPET is compared to maximum voluntary ventilation to determine breathing reserve. Athletes generate large tidal volumes and maximum V_E during exercise may be well in excess of values traditionally observed among nonathletic populations, sometimes in excess of 200 L/min.[72] Athletes frequently will have breathing reserves less than 10% to 15%. In nonathletic populations, these values suggest pathology, but among athletes, they may reflect exceptional effort and supraphysiologic cardiorespiratory performance during exercise.

Exercise economy is an important parameter for endurance athletes. Better economy—that is, a lower VO_2 for any given power output—is advantageous since this translates into the utilization of a lower percentage of VO_{2max} for any given exercise intensity (see **Fig. 1**). Exercise economy likely depends on the power outputs at which an athlete trains.[73] Competitive athletes in particular may be interested in improving exercise economy (ie, lowering the slope of the VO_2: work relationship), which may require training over a wide range of power outputs, for example, a runner training at different speeds.[73]

Training Zones, Exercise Prescriptions, and Critical Power

CPET can be used to prescribe individualized training programs based on several physiologic parameters including HR, workload, VT, and VO_{2max}.[20,71] Generally, 4 zones can be described based on CPET performance (see **Fig. 2**)[20,71,73]:

- Zone 1: Workloads below VT1
- Zone 2: Workloads between VT1 and VT2
- Zone 3: Workloads above VT2 resulting in VO_{2max} at exhaustion
- Zone 4: Maximal effort at workloads allowing for ascertainment of VO_{2max}

Zone 1 training involves prolonged and sustainable exercise with a steady VO_2 and, by definition, is well below VT. This level of effort produces at most, mild fatigue, and for athletes participating in high-intensity interval training, Zone 1 is a recovery zone. Zone 2 training, occurring at greater workloads, still falls below the respiratory compensation point and has been shown to improve VO_2 and lactate concentration during submaximal exercise. VT2 has been established as a key indicator of an athlete's maximal steady state—that is, the exercise intensity above which exercise cannot be sustained

for prolonged periods.[24,74–76] For example, among cyclists, VT2 reliably indicates the maximal intensity that is sustainable during a 30 minute time trial.[77]

Critical power refers to the highest workload that can be achieved with a steady-state lactate concentration and represents a marker of the upper limit of sustainable prolonged exercise.[71,73] Identification of critical power is of particular relevance to endurance athletes, such as marathoners and triathletes, seeking to identify the maximal workload/speed that can be sustained during competition. Zones 3 and 4, by definition, are not sustainable levels of effort and can only be maintained for several minutes based on the fitness and conditioning of the athlete. Zone 3 workloads are in excess of critical power. Athletes exercising in Zone 3 do not achieve a steady state of VO_2 but rather achieve VO_{2max} at the point of exhaustion during the exercise bout. Zone 4 workloads are those that occur at/near VO_{2max} (sometimes called the "red zone," referring to at least 90% of VO_{2max}),[78] and since these very short-term duration workloads are non-sustainable, they are used primarily for high-intensity exercise training.[78]

SUMMARY

A lifelong commitment to exercise leads to cardiac remodeling with alterations in atrial and ventricular structure and function. Exercise testing in athletes may be necessary for many purposes, such as determining whether cardiac remodeling is the result of an athletic heart or due to cardiomyopathy, as well as identifying fitness level and overall functional capacity, and/or establishing training zones. Given their unique training, athletes exhibit several unique physiologic responses to exercise testing, and testing protocols must be tailored appropriately.

CLINICS CARE POINTS

- Cardiopulmonary exercise testing can be helpful for athletes wanting to determine exercise training zones.

- Cardiopulmonary exercise testing is a helpful test to understand causes of exertional symptoms such as lightheadedness, dyspnea, and/or impairments in exercise capacity. This type of test is preferred over a standard exercise tolerance test.

- When completing exercise tests, the specific protocol for testing should be individually tailored to the athlete with all efforts made to replicate an athlete's specific type of exercise.

DISCLOSURE

None.

REFERENCES

1. Master A, Oppenheimer E. A simple exercise tolerance test for circulatory efficiency with standard tables for normal individuals. Am J Med Sci 1929; 177:233–5.
2. Russek HI. Master two-step test in coronary artery disease. J Am Med Assoc 1957;165:1772–5.
3. Moss AJ. Exercise testing. Ann Noninvasive Electrocardiol 2004;9:199–200.
4. Forbes LM, Bull TM, Lahm T, et al. Exercise Testing in the Risk Assessment of Pulmonary Hypertension. Chest 2023;164:736–46.
5. Balady GJ, Ades PA. Exercise Physiology and Exercise Electrocardiographic Testing. In: Libby P, Bonow RO, Mann DL, et al, editors. Braunwald's heart disease: a textbook of cardiovascular medicine. 12th edition. Philadelphia, PA: Elsevier; 2022. p. 175–95.
6. Wasfy MM. CPET: Basis of Performance & Interpretation. Care of the Athletic Heart 2023.
7. Balady GJ, Arena R, Sietsema K, et al, American Heart Association Exercise CR, Prevention Committee of the Council on Clinical C, Council on E, Prevention, Council on Peripheral Vascular D, Interdisciplinary Council on Quality of C and Outcomes R. Clinician's Guide to cardiopulmonary exercise testing in adults: a scientific statement from the American Heart Association. Circulation 2010;122: 191–225.
8. Ommen SR, Mital S, Burke MA, et al. 2020 AHA/ ACC Guideline for the Diagnosis and Treatment of Patients With Hypertrophic Cardiomyopathy: A Report of the American College of Cardiology/ American Heart Association Joint Committee on Clinical Practice Guidelines. Circulation 2020;142: e558–631.
9. Lorenz DS, Reiman MP, Lehecka BJ, et al. What performance characteristics determine elite versus nonelite athletes in the same sport? Sports Health 2013;5:542–7.
10. Swann C, Moran A, Piggott D. Defining elite athletes: Issues in the study of expert performance in sport psychology. Psychol Sport Exerc 2015;16:3–14.
11. Levine BD, Baggish AL, Kovacs RJ, et al, Arrhythmias Committee of Council on Clinical Cardiology CoCDiY-CoC, Stroke Nursing CoFG, Translational B and American College of C. Eligibility and Disqualification Recommendations for Competitive Athletes With Cardiovascular Abnormalities: Task Force 1: Classification of Sports: Dynamic, Static, and Impact: A Scientific Statement From the American Heart Association and American College of Cardiology. Circulation 2015;132:e262–6.
12. Edward JA, Cornwell WK. Impact of Exercise on Cerebrovascular Physiology and Risk of Stroke. Stroke 2022;53:2404–10.
13. Dos Santos M, Ferrari G, Lee DH, et al. Association of the "Weekend Warrior" and Other Leisure-time Physical Activity Patterns With All-Cause and Cause-Specific Mortality: A Nationwide Cohort Study. JAMA Intern Med 2022;182:840–8.
14. Huang J, McDonnell BJ, Lawley JS, et al. Impact of Mechanical Circulatory Support on Exercise Capacity in Patients with Advanced Heart Failure. Exerc Sport Sci Rev 2022;50:222–9.
15. Treacher DF, Leach RM. ABC of Oxygen. Oxygen transport - 1. Basic Principles. Britich Medical Journal 1998;317:1302–6.
16. Sarma S, Levine B. Exercise Physiology for the Clinician. Exercise and Sports Cardiology, vol. 1. 2nd edition. Singapore: World Scientific Publishing Europe Ltd; 2018. p. 23–62.
17. Rowell LB. Human circulation: regulation during physical stress. 1st Edition. New York: Oxford Univesrity Press; 1986.
18. Proctor DN, Beck KC, Shen PH, et al. Influence of age and gender on cardiac output- Vo2 relationships during submaximal cycle ergometry. J Appl Physiol 1998;84:599–605.
19. Gledhill N, Cox D, Jamnik R. Endurance athletes' stroke volume does not plateau: major advantage is diastolic function. Med Sci Sports Exerc 1994; 26:1116–21.
20. Mazaheri R, Schmied C, Niederseer D, et al. Cardiopulmonary Exercise Test Parameters in Athletic Population: A Review. J Clin Med 2021;10:5073.
21. van Ingen Schenau GJ, Cavanagh PR. Power equations in endurance sports. J Biomech 1990;23:865–81.
22. Lucia A, Sanchez O, Carvajal A, et al. Analysis of the aerobic-anaerobic transition in elite cyclists during incremental exercise with the use of electromyography. Br J Sports Med 1999;33:178–85.
23. Lucia A, Hoyos J, Perez M, et al. Heart rate and performance parameters in elite cyclists: a longitudinal study. Med Sci Sports Exerc 2000;32:1777–82.
24. Cerezuela-Espejo V, Courel-IBanez J, MOran-Navarro R, et al. The relationship between lactate and ventilatory thresholds in runners - validity and reliability of exercise test performance parameters. Front Physiol 2018;9. https://doi.org/10.3389/fphys.2018.01320.
25. Brooks GA. Anaerobic threshold: review of the concept and directions for future research. Med Sci Sports Exerc 1985;17:22–34.
26. Conconi F, Grazzi G, Casoni I, et al. The Conconi test: Methodology after 12 years of application. Int J Sports Med 1996;17:509–19.
27. Beaudry R, Haykowsky MJ, Baggish A, et al. A Modern Definition of the Athlete's Heart-for Research and the Clinic. Cardiol Clin 2016;34:507–14.

28. Prior DL, La Gerche A. The athlete's heart. Heart 2012;98:947–55.

29. Morganroth J, Maron BJ, Henry WL, et al. Comparative Left Ventricular Dimensions in Trained Athletes. Ann Intern Med 1975;82:802–6.

30. Levine BD, Baggish AL, Kovacs RJ, et al. Eligibility and Disqualification Recommendations for Competitive Athletes With Cardiovascular Abnormalities: Task Force 1: Classification of Sports: Dynamic, Static, and Impact. J Am Coll Cardiol 2015;66:2350–5.

31. Fagard RH. Athlete's heart: a meta-analysis of the echocardiographic experience. Int J Sports Med 1996;17(Suppl 3):S140–4.

32. Roy A, Doyon M, Dumesnil JG, et al. Endurance vs. strength training - comparison of cardiac structures using normal predicted values. J Appl Physiol 1988; 64:2552–7.

33. Pluim BM, Zwinderman AH, van der Laarse A, et al. The Athlete's Heart. A Meta-Analysis of Cardiac Structure and Function. Circulation 1999;100:336–44.

34. Weiner RB, Baggish AL. Exercise-induced cardiac remodeling. Prog Cardiovasc Dis 2012;54:380–6.

35. Scharhag J, Schneider G, Urhausen A, et al. Athlete's heart: right and left ventricular mass and function in male endurance athletes and untrained individuals determined by magnetic resonance imaging. J Am Coll Cardiol 2002;40:1856–63.

36. Cornwell WK, Buttrick P. Mechanobiology of exercise-induced cardiac remodeling in health and disease. Cardiac Mechanobiology in Physiology in Health and Disease, vol 1. 1st edition. Cham Switzerland: Springer; 2023. p. 211–28.

37. D'Andrea A, Riegler L, Golia E, et al. Range of right heart measurements in top-level athletes: the training impact. Int J Cardiol 2013;164:48–57.

38. Kim JH, Noseworthy PA, McCarty D, et al. Significance of electrocardiographic right bundle branch block in trained athletes. Am J Cardiol 2011;107: 1083–9.

39. Scharf M, Brem MH, Wilhelm M, et al. Cardiac magnetic resonance assessment of left and right ventricular morphologic and functional adaptations in professional soccer players. Am Heart J 2010;159: 911–8.

40. Scharhag J, Schneider G, Urhausen A, et al. Athlete's heart: right and left ventricular mass and function in male endurance athletes and untrained individuals determined by magnetic resonance imaging. J Am Coll Cardiol 2002;40:1856–63.

41. Henriksen E, Landelius J, Wesslen L, et al. Echocardiographic right and left ventricular measurements in male elite endurance athletes. Eur Heart J 1996; 17:1121–8.

42. Baggish AL, Wang F, Weiner RB, et al. Training-specific changes in cardiac structure and function: a prospective and longitudinal assessment of competitive athletes. J Appl Physiol (1985) 2008;104:1121–8.

43. Cornwell WK, Tran T, Cerbin L, et al. New insights into resting and exertional right ventricular performance in the healthy heart through real-time pressure-volume analysis. J Physiol 2020;598:2575–87.

44. Edward J, Banchs J, Parker H, et al. Right ventricular function across the spectrum of health and disease. Heart 2023;109:349–55.

45. La Gerche A, Heidbuchel H, Burns AT, et al. Disproportionate exercise load and remodeling of the athlete's right ventricle. Med Sci Sports Exerc 2011;43: 974–81.

46. La Gerche A, Burns AT, Mooney DJ, et al. Exercise-induced right ventricular dysfunction and structural remodelling in endurance athletes. Eur Heart J 2012;33:998–1006.

47. Oxborough D, Shave R, Warburton D, et al. Dilatation and dysfunction of the right ventricle immediately after ultraendurance exercise: exploratory insights from conventional two-dimensional and speckle tracking echocardiography. Circ Cardiovasc Imaging 2011;4:253–63.

48. La Gerche A, Connelly KA, Mooney DJ, et al. Biochemical and functional abnormalities of left and right ventricular function after ultra-endurance exercise. Heart 2008;94:860–6.

49. Elliott AD, La Gerche A. The right ventricle following prolonged endurance exercise: are we overlooking the more important side of the heart? A meta-analysis. Br J Sports Med 2015;49:724–9.

50. Edward JA, Cerbin LP, Groves DW, et al. Right Ventricular Dysfunction During Endurance Exercise as Determined by Pressure-Volume Analysis. JACC (J Am Coll Cardiol): Case Reports 2022;4:1435–8.

51. Bhella PS, Hastings JL, Fujimoto N, et al. Impact of lifelong exercise "dose" on left ventricular compliance and distensibility. J Am Coll Cardiol 2014;64: 1257–66.

52. Howden EJ, Sarma S, Lawley JS, et al. Reversing the Cardiac Effects of Sedentary Aging in Middle Age-A Randomized Controlled Trial: Implications For Heart Failure Prevention. Circulation 2018;137: 1549–60.

53. Pelliccia A, Maron BJ, Di Paolo FM, et al. Prevalence and clinical significance of left atrial remodeling in competitive athletes. J Am Coll Cardiol 2005;46: 690–6.

54. Jin MN, Yang PS, Song C, et al. Physical Activity and Risk of Atrial Fibrillation: A Nationwide Cohort Study in General Population. Sci Rep 2019;9:13270.

55. Malmo V, Nes BM, Amundsen BH, et al. Aerobic Interval Training Reduces the Burden of Atrial Fibrillation in the Short Term: A Randomized Trial. Circulation 2016;133:466–73.

56. Mozaffarian D, Furberg CD, Psaty BM, et al. Physical activity and incidence of atrial fibrillation in older adults: the cardiovascular health study. Circulation 2008;118:800–7.

57. Aizer A, Giaziano JM, Cook NR, et al. Relation of Vigorous Exercise Risk to Risk of Atrial Fibrillation. Am J Cardiol 2009;103:1572–7.

58. Thelle DS, Selmer R, Gjesdal K, et al. Resrting heart rate and physical activity as risk factors for lone atrial fibrillation: a prosepctive study of 309,540 men and women. Heart 2013;99:1713.

59. Drca N, Wolk A, Jensen-Urstad M, et al. Atrial fibrillation is associated with different levels of physical activity levels at different ages in men. Heart 2014; 100:1043–9.

60. Andersen K, Farahmand B, Ahlbom A, et al. Risk of arrhythmias in 52 755 long-distance cross-country skiers: a cohort study. Eur Heart J 2013;34:3624–31.

61. Guasch E, Mont L, Sitges M. Mechanisms of atrial fibrillation in athletes: what we know and what we do not know. Neth Heart J 2018;26:133–45.

62. Trivedi SJ, Claessen G, Stefani L, et al. Differing mechanisms of atrial fibrillation in athletes and non-athletes: alterations in atrial structure and function. Eur Heart J Cardiovasc Imaging 2020;21: 1374–83.

63. Wilhelm M, Roten L, Tanner H, et al. Atrial remodeling, autonomic tone, and lifetime training hours in nonelite athletes. Am J Cardiol 2011;108:580–5.

64. Kasapis C, Thompson PD. The effects of physical activity on serum C-reactive protein and inflammatory markers: a systematic review. J Am Coll Cardiol 2005;45:1563–9.

65. La Gerche A, Inder WJ, Roberts TJ, et al. Relationship between Inflammatory Cytokines and Indices of Cardiac Dysfunction following Intense Endurance Exercise. PLoS One 2015;10:e0130031.

66. Svedberg N, Sundstrom J, James S, et al. Long-Term Incidence of Atrial Fibrillation and Stroke Among Cross-Country Skiers. Circulation 2019;140: 910–20.

67. La Gerche A, Heidbuchel H. Can intensive exercise harm the heart? You can get too much of a good thing. Circulation 2014;130:992–1002.

68. Parizher G, Emery MS. Exercise Stress Testing in Athletes. Clin Sports Med 2022;41:441–54.

69. Kang J, Chaloupka EC, Mastrangelo MA, et al. Physiological comparisons among three maximal treadmill exercise protocols in trained and untrained individuals. Eur J Appl Physiol 2001;84:291–5.

70. Jain M, Nkonde C, Lin BA, et al. 85% of maximal age-predicted heart rate is not a valid endpoint for exercise treadmill testing. J Nucl Cardiol 2011;18: 1026–35.

71. Mezzani A, Hamm LF, Jones AM, et al. Aerobic exercise intensity assessment and prescription in cardiac rehabilitation: a joint position statement of the European Association for Cardiovascular Prevention and Rehabilitation, the American Association of Cardiovascular and Pulmonary Rehabilitation and the Canadian Association of Cardiac Rehabilitation. Eur J Prev Cardiol 2013;20:442–67.

72. Hanson JS. Maximal exercise performance in members of the US Nordic Ski Team. J Appl Physiol 1973; 35:592–5.

73. Jones AM, Carter HH. The effect of endurance training on parameters of aerobic fitness. Sports Med 2000;29:373–86.

74. Ghosh AK. Anaerobic Threshold: Its Concept and Role in Endurance Sport. Malays J Med Sci 2004; 11:24–36.

75. Lanferdini FJ, Silva ES, Machado E, et al. Physiological Predictors of Maximal Incremental Running Performance. Front Physiol 2020;11:979.

76. Bentley DJ, Newell J, Bishop D. Incremental Exercise Test Design and Analysis. Implications for Performance Diagnostics in Endurance Athletes. Sports Med 2007;37:575–86.

77. Perrey S, Grappe F, Girard A, et al. Physiological and Metabolic Responses of Triathletes to a Simulated 30-min Time-Trial in Cycling at Self-Selected Intensity. Int J Sports Med 2003;24:138–43.

78. Buchheit M, Laursen PB. High-intensity interval training, solutions to the programming puzzle: Part I: cardiopulmonary emphasis. Sports Med 2013;43: 313–38.

Exercise Hemodynamics in Heart Failure with Preserved Ejection Fraction

Satyam Sarma, MD[a,b],*

KEYWORDS

- HFpEF • Exercise • Hemodynamics • Pulmonary capillary wedge pressure

KEY POINTS

- Pulmonary capillary wedge pressure (PCWP) measures are influenced by pleural pressures. In patients with obesity, pleural pressures can be positive even under resting circumstances. As prevalence of obesity increases among patients with heart failure with preserved ejection fraction (HFpEF), measuring and reporting resting and exercise PCWP in isolation may overestimate cardiopulmonary hemodynamics.
- PCWP/cardiac output slopes can be useful in aiding diagnosis of HFpEF in patients with low exercise capacity but should be interpreted with caution. Patients at risk for HFpEF but without overt heart failure may present with an elevated slope. Similarly, some patients with HFpEF may have a blunted slope emphasizing the importance of multi-modal diagnosis for HFpEF including symptoms, echocardiography, biomarker, and hemodynamic data.
- An elevated V-wave in the setting of poor left atrial compliance represents a particularly malignant form of HFpEF with low diffusing capacity of the lungs for carbon monoxide and elevated pulmonary pressures.

INTRODUCTION

Heart failure with preserved ejection, or HFpEF, remains a challenging condition to diagnose and treat. Exercise or exertional intolerance is a dominant symptom for many patients. While metabolic therapies such as sodium/glucose transporter 2 inhibitors[1,2] and glucagon like peptide-1 receptor agonists[3] have shown promise in reducing heart failure hospitalization and quality of life, strategies to improve exercise capacity have had variable effects. As the number of patients with HFpEF is projected to increase in the coming decades from an aging population suffering from higher rates of obesity and diabetes, better understanding of the physiologic mechanisms underlying poor exercise tolerance, specifically exercise hemodynamics, may inform new therapeutic approaches. This review will discuss the utility of exercise hemodynamics under both diagnostic and prognostic circumstances and highlight challenges associated with making and interpreting measures taken during exercise.

PULMONARY CAPILLARY WEDGE PRESSURE

HFpEF is a clinical diagnosis. The presence of heart failure symptoms (eg, orthopnea, paroxysmal nocturnal dyspnea, lower extremity edema) and elevated plasma natriuretic peptide levels in conjunction with a preserved ejection fraction is sufficient for diagnosis. Unfortunately, many common comorbid conditions (eg, obesity, advanced age, obstructive sleep apnea) can

Funding Information: National Institutes of Health 1P01HL137630; American Heart Association Career Development Award.
a Department of Internal Medicine, University of Texas Southwestern Medical Center, Dallas, TX, USA;
b Institute for Exercise and Environmental Medicine, Texas Health Presbyterian Hospital Dallas, Dallas, TX, USA
* 7232 Greenville Avenue, Suite 435, Dallas, TX 75231.
E-mail address: Satyam.Sarma@UTSouthwestern.edu

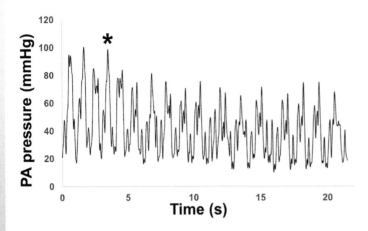

Fig. 1. Example of the rapid drop in pulmonary pressures after stopping exercise in a patient with heart failure with preserved ejection fraction (HFpEF). The asterisk denotes when exercise was stopped. Pressures return to baseline within approximately 10 seconds.

confound these criteria and objective evidence for elevated left ventricular filling pressures can be useful to confirm or refute diagnosis. Right heart catheterization therefore is the gold standard in diagnosing HFpEF. A supine resting pulmonary capillary wedge pressure (PCWP) greater than 15 mm Hg or supine exercise peak PCWP greater than 25 mm Hg is considered diagnostic.[4]

From a cardiac perspective, increases in PCWP with exercise are a result of low LV compliance (ie, increased stiffness) and impaired ventricular relaxation. There are few readily available clinical tools that can accurately characterize left ventricular (LV) stiffness and relaxation. Instead, exercise PCWP is useful as a surrogate for LV diastolic dysfunction and in addition to diagnostic utility, can also provide important prognostic information. In a study of 355 patients with HFpEF,[5] higher resting and exercise PCWP was associated with increased mortality. In patients with both elevated resting and exercise PCWP, mortality was nearly 5 times higher than those with normal pressures. Even in patients with normal resting pressures but elevated exercise PCWP had an over 2-fold higher rate of mortality. It should be noted that high PCWP during exercise is not a marker of pulmonary congestion or acute heart failure. In the upright position, the rapid rise of pressures at the onset of exertion quickly returns back to baseline once exercise is stopped (**Fig. 1**). The short duration of exercise is insufficient to cause pulmonary congestion, although in the supine position, where pressures are higher, this has been observed.[6,7] Thus, the main significance of an elevated PCWP is identifying patients who are likely to have higher LV stiffness and slowed relaxation.

An important question is whether PCWP should be measured at end-expiration or during spontaneous respiration. Inter-thoracic pressures can have significant effects on cardiopulmonary pressures. Throughout the respiratory cycle, recoil from lung tissue opposes the chest wall. Fluctuation in these forces can change pleural pressures which in turn exert effects on PCWP. Under resting conditions, end-expiration occurs at functional residual capacity (FRC), a lung volume at which pleural pressures are 0 as positive recoil pressures from forces generated by lung compliance are balanced by negative pressures form chest wall compliance. Measuring pressures at end-expiration minimizes the effects of respiratory system influence. These assumptions unfortunately do not hold true in patients with obesity or respiratory disease.[8] Whether by excess thoracic mass in obesity or hyperinflation and air trapping in chronic obstructive pulmonary disease, pleural pressures (through changes in lung and chest wall compliance) can be positive at FRC, leading to overestimation of PCWP. During exercise, effects of pleural pressure swings from inspiration to expiration can be further amplified.[9]

There are a few strategies to mitigate the effects of respiratory swings on PCWP measures during exercise. These approaches include placing an esophageal balloon to allow for real-time correction of pleural pressures, calculating LV transmural pressure from PCWP and central venous pressures, averaging PCWP across several respiratory cycles, or measuring PCWP during spontaneous or controlled end-expiration breath holds. Measuring and adjusting for pleural and to a less extent right atrial pressures, can be useful in estimating LV transmural pressures. The LV transmural pressure represents the "net" filling pressure after subtracting external compression pressures from the pleura and provides a more accurate assessment of cardiac filling in the face of large respiratory pressure swings (**Fig. 2**). In the absence of esophageal balloon manometry for pleural pressures, right atrial pressures can also

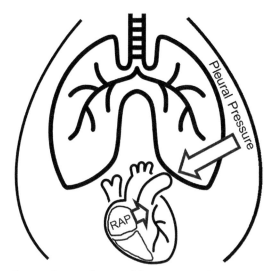

Fig. 2. Schema of external forces upon left ventricular filling. Chronic conditions such as obesity and respiratory diseases can cause pleural pressures to be elevated even under resting conditions. These compressive forces from the pleura can increase pulmonary pressures, including pulmonary capillary wedge pressure. Similarly, right atrial pressures (RAP) can be elevated in the setting of high pericardial pressures (eg, constriction) or right ventricular dysfunction. Because of shared space within the pericardium, elevated right-sided pressures can exert compressive effects on left ventricular filling.

be used to estimate LV transmural pressures.[10] A key limitation with these methods is that abnormal thresholds at rest or during exercise have not been established.

Instead, averaging across multiple respiratory cycles or measuring pressures at end-expiration is more common clinically as established thresholds exist. For patients who cannot perform a breath hold at end-expiration during exercise, an average of several spontaneous end-expiratory breaths be used (**Fig. 3**). As noted earlier, a resting PCWP greater than 15 mm Hg or an exercise peak PCWP greater than 25 mm Hg is considered diagnostic for HFpEF.[4] An important point is that these thresholds are for supine exercise and can be confounded by changes in respiratory system compliance from obesity or respiratory diseases. This can increase pleural pressure which in turn can increase PCWP. The effects are magnified during exercise when changes in pleural pressure are greatest. Averaging across several breaths does mitigate the dynamic swings in pleural pressures but does not account for low respiratory system compliance.

While lung compliance cannot be easily changed, 1 way to minimize the effects of chest wall compliance is to shift exercise from supine to upright. In contrast to the supine position where the entire weight of chest and abdominal fat is distributed directly onto the thorax, the upright posture shifts majority of the compressive forces away from these compartments. In patients with obesity, changing from being upright to lying supine results in larger increases in intra-thoracic pressures compared to normal weight individuals.[11] In a cohort of obese patients with pulmonary hypertension, the compressive effects from thoracic pressure measured by an esophageal balloon were higher in the supine compared to seated positions by an average of 9 mm Hg at end-expiration.[12] Adjusting for intra-thoracic pressure, the transmural or adjusted PCWP decreased by 14 mm Hg in the supine position and 5 mm Hg when upright. Thus, to a significant degree, elevated PCWP in the supine position and to a lesser degree in the upright position was due to constraining or compressive effects from high intra-thoracic or pleural pressure. Exercising in the upright position may provide a more accurate assessment of "true" exercise pressures, particularly in those who are obese. While clinical thresholds for upright exercise are not established, using similar supine criteria of peak PCWP greater than 25 mm Hg or a peak greater than 20 mm Hg to account for lower starting upright pressures is reasonable.[13]

These issues highlight the challenges of interpreting pressures during exercise. While invasive exercise hemodynamics is not particularly difficult technically, understanding the factors that impact cardiopulmonary pressures becomes increasingly important. As the prevalence of obesity and morbid/super-obesity increases among patients with HFpEF, measuring and reporting resting and exercise PCWP in isolation may overestimate cardiopulmonary hemodynamics. Rather, strategies that contextualize PCWP changes during exercise may provide a more accurate understanding of patients' exercise hemodynamics.

CARDIAC OUTPUT PRESSURE SLOPES

As described in the previous section, there are many potential confounding factors in interpreting exercise PCWP in isolation. One scenario not addressed is patients who meet clinical criteria for heart failure but have a non-diagnostic exercise hemodynamic profile. Patients who are limited by frailty, orthopedic injuries may not be able to exercise at work rate sufficient to increase cardiac output and venous return and fail to reach a peak PCWP of 25 mm Hg. Normalizing PCWP to cardiac output (>2 mm Hg/L/min)[14] as a surrogate for venous return may better identify these patients.[15]

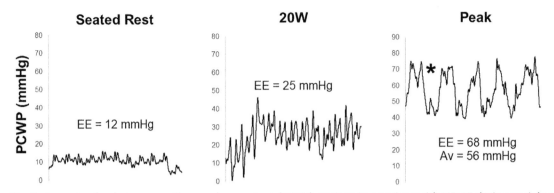

Fig. 3. Example of pulmonary capillary wedge pressure (PCWP) tracings in a patient with HFpEF during upright rest, 20 W of seated cycle exercise and peak exercise. At rest and 20 W, patient was able to perform voluntary breath holds at end-expiration (EE). At peak exercise, PCWP was measured as both spontaneous EE breaths (high plateau phase; *asterisk*) and an average across 5 cardiac cycles. For EE measures, an average of each spontaneous EE pressure was taken.

Alternatively, PCWP/cardiac output slope can also be used to exclude the diagnosis of HFpEF from patients who have high exercise PCWP arising from a high-output state (eg, trained, older person; anemia).

Guyton's venous return curves describe the relationship between venous return and cardiac output. Under resting conditions, increased venous return leads to increases in cardiac output as a function of increased LV end-diastolic volume (EDV). With exercise, as non-exercising vascular beds constrict, there is a shift toward larger effective circulating blood volume which in turn raises venous pressures.[16] In a healthy heart, the resultant increase in LV EDV from higher venous pressures leads to higher stroke volume and cardiac output via Starling mechanisms. As exercise intensity increases, further rises in cardiac output are from increases in heart rate as changes in stroke volume plateaus.[17] Thus, the PCWP/cardiac output slope captures 2 prominent features of exercise hemodynamics in HFpEF—rapid and large increases in PCWP in the numerator and blunted heart rate/SV response in the denominator.[18] Exercise cardiac output will be discussed in more detail later.

It should be noted that a low cardiac output and hyperdynamic PCWP response to exercise may also be present prior to the diagnosis of overt HFpEF. In a study of 110 patients with dyspnea of unexplained etiology,[14] a PCWP/cardiac output slope greater than 2 mm Hg/L/min was associated with over 3-fold higher rates for the composite end point of future heart failure hospitalization, cardiovascular death, or development of PCWP greater than 15 mm Hg. These results suggest abnormal hemodynamic responses to exercise can be useful for identifying those at-risk for, or stage B, heart failure. This does raise the possibility of over-diagnosing HFpEF if PCWP/cardiac output slope is the sole determining feature and emphasizes

that HFpEF is a clinical diagnosis and as highlighted earlier in the review.

Alternatively, a low PCWP/cardiac output slope does not necessarily rule out HFpEF. In a study of 563 patients with HFpEF diagnosed on basis of supine invasive hemodynamic (rest PCWP > 15 mm Hg or exercise PCWP > 25 mm Hg), 70 patients (12%) had slopes less than 2 mm Hg/L/min despite elevated exercise PCWP.[19] These patients, compared to the overall HFpEF cohort were more obese (average body mass index [BMI] 34.0 vs 32.4 kg/m^2), had lower peak exercise PCWP (28 vs 32 mm Hg), higher exercise cardiac output (12.3 vs 9.1 L/min) but had similar resting PCWP (17 vs 16 mm Hg), E/e' (13 vs 13), e' (7 vs 8 cm/s), and tricuspid regurgitant velocities (2.6 vs 2.5 m/s). As invasive exercise testing is not routinely performed clinically, it would be difficult to discern differences in those with and without slopes greater than 2 based on resting hemodynamic and diastolic function parameters alone. It is unclear then what low PCWP/cardiac output slopes in patients with HFpEF represent. Is it an effect of hyperdynamic cardiac output response during exercise common in patients with obesity and HFpEF[20] or patients with HFpEF for whom exercise intolerance is not attributable to a cardiac limitation[21]? Further studies are needed to understand the clinical significance and physiologic mechanism of low PCWP/cardiac output slope in HFpEF.

PULMONARY CAPILLARY WEDGE PRESSURE AND OUTCOMES

All in all, exercise hemodynamics is useful for diagnosing, prognosing, and potentially phenotyping patients with HFpEF. While PCWP and PCWP/cardiac output thresholds are useful diagnostically, these are continuous variables and there is likely important prognostic information along the

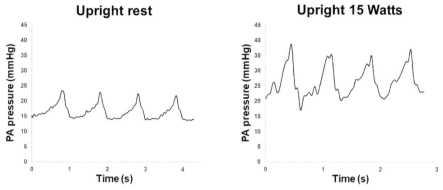

Fig. 4. Example of V-waves from a pulmonary capillary wedge pressure tracing in a patient with HFpEF. The patient had a history of multiple atrial fibrillation ablations and was in atrial flutter at time of exercise hemodynamic measures. No apparent A-wave can be seen. At rest, V-waves are approximately 22 mm Hg. With light exercise, V-waves increase to 35 mm Hg.

spectrum of these individual patient responses. In addition, in patients with pulmonary venous disease, mitral valve disorders, and left atrial dysfunction (eg, chronic atrial fibrillation, multiple left atrial ablations, infiltrative myopathy etc), PCWP is not an accurate surrogate of left ventricular filling pressure. Patients with these conditions may have an elevated PCWP due primarily to large V-waves (**Fig. 4**). With exercise, the height of the V-wave can reach over 60 mm Hg. Since the V-wave represents retrograde pressure transmitted from the left atrium into the pulmonary arteries, potentially leading to paradoxically higher PCWP than pulmonary artery diastolic pressure, these effects are more likely to impact pulmonary rather than cardiac function. In a study of 106 patients with HFpEF without severe valvular disease undergoing simultaneous left heart and pulmonary pressure measurements,[22] PCWP averaged across several cardiac cycles was more strongly associated with the primary outcome of heart failure hospitalization and cardiovascular death than LV end-diastolic pressure. Patients with higher PCWP to LVEDP gradients had lower diffusing capacity of the lungs for carbon monoxide (DLCO), and lower capillary partial pressure of oxygen and carbon dioxide. In multi-variable regression, only DLCO was significantly associated with a larger PCWP-LVEDP gradient suggesting impairments in pulmonary gas exchange. Although V-waves were not explicitly reported as the entirety of the PCWP waveform was averaged across several cardiac cycles, in the absence of severe valvular disease, the large PCWP-LVEDP gradients were likely a result of left atrial dysfunction (stiffness and/or severe dilation).

The bidirectional nature of PCWP on both cardiac and pulmonary function may be useful in understanding the elevated risk associated with atrial fibrillation (AF) and HFpEF. AF is linked to an atrial myopathy characterized by increased LA stiffness and size.[23] The degree of this myopathy is proportional to AF severity (eg, paroxysmal vs permanent). In a study of 97 patients with HFpEF and AF compared to 181 patients with HFpEF without AF, AF was associated with increased LA stiffness, higher pulmonary vascular resistance, higher pulmonary pressures, and higher V wave.[24] Patients with AF had nearly 2 times greater 10-year mortality than those without AF. That the magnitude of V-wave elevation was proportional to AF severity, suggests this component of the PCWP waveform may be as important prognostically as an elevated exercise PCWP or PCWP/cardiac output slope. The mechanisms mediating risks associated with chronically elevated V-wave are likely attributable to pulmonary vascular remodeling and resistance, increased right ventricular dysfunction, and respiratory gas exchange impairments.

Thus, the relationship between PCWP, cardiac output, pulmonary function, and right-sided dysfunction are all intertwined. To appreciate the hemodynamic profile of a patient with HFpEF requires understanding all 3 components to PCWP—the absolute value at rest and changes with exercise, the ratio of PCWP to cardiac output response during exercise, and the V-wave. Each highlights a unique aspect of exercise hemodynamic response in HFpEF and eventually may be used to guide personalized therapies.

CARDIAC OUTPUT EXERCISE RESPONSE IN HEART FAILURE WITH PRESERVED EJECTION FRACTION

The relationship between cardiac output and hemodynamics mimics the apocryphal chicken and egg.

Abnormalities in hemodynamic response can affect cardiac responses during exercise and vice versa. Specifically, increases in stroke volume during exercise depend on PCWP and efficiency of Starling mechanisms. As shown in **Fig. 2**, ventricular filling does not occur in isolation and reflects on net pressures exerted on the myocardium. As noted earlier, pleural pressures can exert pressures on structures within the thorax. Pressure exerted on the lungs is equally exerted on the heart such that net transmural pressure responsible for cardiac filling is unaffected. Similarly, disproportionate increases in right-sided cardiac pressures from right ventricular dysfunction can also restrict left ventricular filling. Using right atrial pressure (RAP) as a surrogate for right-sided and pericardial pressures, the intrinsic cardiac transmural pressure can be calculated as PCWP− RAP. Thus, the net pressure dictating LV filling is PCWP− RAP−pleural pressure.

Similarly, increases in cardiac output can lead to increased cardiopulmonary pressures. As cardiac output increases with exercise, pressures increase even in healthy individuals.[25] With increased ventricular and vascular stiffening, such as with sedentary aging, cardiopulmonary pressures are higher for similar relative exercise intensities as higher venous returns lead to higher pressures in a low compliance ventricle.[26] While the PCWP/cardiac output slope can be useful to understand these relationships, in instances where the slope is very elevated, it is necessary to understand whether the primary factor driving this ratio is a low exercise cardiac output response.

Defining a normal cardiac output response to exercise requires understanding the metabolic demands placed on the body. As an example, an exercise cardiac output of 12 L/min could be considered normal, high, or low if the exercise work rate was 150 W, 20 W, or 250 W, respectively. Under normal muscle metabolic function, increases in cardiac output are proportional to metabolic oxidative capacity such that at higher exercise intensities, more oxygen needs to be delivered to the exercising muscle. As an extreme example, patients with mitochondrial myopathies who have defects in oxidative phosphorylation can have hyper-dynamic cardiac output responses to exercise as the exercising muscle demands more oxygen despite impairments in aerobic respiration.[27] As the vast majority of Vo_2 increases with exercise are from increased muscle metabolic activity, normalizing cardiac output to Vo_2 can be useful in determining if an exercise cardiac output is appropriate or inappropriate for a given exercise intensity. A cardiac output/Vo_2 slope of 5 to 6 is considered normal across age, sex, and fitness levels.[28,29] Patients with heart failure with reduced ejection fraction have blunted or low cardiac output/Vo_2 slopes.[30]

There is considerable variability in cardiac output/Vo_2 slopes in patients with HFpEF with studies suggesting both blunted[31] and hyperdynamic cardiac output responses.[21,32] The variability may depend on body position during exercise. Resting cardiac output is higher in the supine than upright position and for the same resting metabolism, leads to a higher starting point for the slope calculation.[33] This in turn can shift the slope lower. In addition, there is likely to intersubject variability and group differences may also reflect differences in patient selection. Some patients with HFpEF may have blunted stroke volume reserve and cardiac output during exercise. Conversely, patients may have capillary oxygen diffusion impairments which lead to decreased oxidative capacity.[21,32] The natural variability in patient responses may be a useful phenotyping strategy to identify patients with HFpEF who are more likely to be cardiac or peripherally limited.

In conclusion, exercise hemodynamics serves several key diagnostic, prognostic, and phenotypic purposes in patients with HFpEF. While measurements are relatively to perform, interpreting changes in cardiopulmonary pressures with exercise requires careful consideration of body position, effects of external compressive forces on pressure measurements, and contextualization of hemodynamics responses to relative changes in cardiac output and metabolic demand. In addition, focusing on particularly high-risk hemodynamic features (eg, presence of large V waves, low cardiac output/Vo_2 slopes) may be useful to identify patients requiring more intensive management of their HFpEF.

CLINICS CARE POINTS

- HFpEF is first and foremost a clinical diagnosis and requires the presence of heart failure symptoms. Diagnostic testing can be useful in confirming diagnosis but should be used in caution in patients without classic heart failure symptoms (eg, orthopnea, paroxysmal nocturnal dyspnea) or heart failure hospitalizations.

- Resting PCWP greater than 15 mm Hg or exercise PCWP greater than 25 mm Hg is considered diagnostic for HFpEF.

- PCWP/cardiac output slope greater than 2 mm Hg/L/min during exercise can also be diagnostic for patients with HFpEF, particularly those with low exercise capacity.

- PCWP/cardiac output slopes can also detect those "at-risk" for HFpEF and should be corroborated with other clinical and laboratory findings to confirm HFpEF diagnosis.
- Normalizing cardiac output to metabolic demand (Vo_2) during exercise is necessary to interpret appropriateness of cardiac output exercise response. A cardiac output/Vo_2 slope of 5 to 6 is considered normal.

DISCLOSURE

The author has nothing to disclose.

REFERENCES

1. Anker SD, Butler J, Filippatos G, et al. Empagliflozin in heart failure with a preserved ejection fraction. N Engl J Med 2021;385(16):1451–61.
2. Borlaug BA, Reddy YNV, Braun A, et al. Cardiac and metabolic effects of dapagliflozin in heart failure with preserved ejection fraction: the CAMEO-DAPA trial. Circulation 2023. https://doi.org/10.1161/CIRCULATIONAHA.123.065134.
3. Kosiborod MN, Abildstrom SZ, Borlaug BA, et al. Semaglutide in patients with heart failure with preserved ejection fraction and obesity. N Engl J Med 2023. https://doi.org/10.1056/NEJMoa2306963.
4. Pieske B, Tschope C, de Boer RA, et al. How to diagnose heart failure with preserved ejection fraction: the HFA-PEFF diagnostic algorithm: a consensus recommendation from the Heart Failure Association (HFA) of the European Society of Cardiology (ESC). Eur Heart J 2019;40(40):3297–317.
5. Dorfs S, Zeh W, Hochholzer W, et al. Pulmonary capillary wedge pressure during exercise and long-term mortality in patients with suspected heart failure with preserved ejection fraction. Eur Heart J 2014;35(44):3103–12.
6. Thompson RB, Chow K, Pagano JJ, et al. Quantification of lung water in heart failure using cardiovascular magnetic resonance imaging. J Cardiovasc Magn Reson 2019;21(1):58.
7. Reddy YNV, Obokata M, Wiley B, et al. The haemodynamic basis of lung congestion during exercise in heart failure with preserved ejection fraction. Eur Heart J 2019;40(45):3721–30.
8. Behazin N, Jones SB, Cohen RI, et al. Respiratory restriction and elevated pleural and esophageal pressures in morbid obesity. J Appl Physiol (1985) 2010;108(1):212–8.
9. Boerrigter BG, Waxman AB, Westerhof N, et al. Measuring central pulmonary pressures during exercise in COPD: how to cope with respiratory effects. Eur Respir J 2014;43(5):1316–25.
10. Smiseth OA, Refsum H, Tyberg JV. Pericardial pressure assessed by right atrial pressure: a basis for calculation of left ventricular transmural pressure. Am Heart J 1984;108(3 Pt 1):603–5.
11. Steier J, Lunt A, Hart N, et al. Observational study of the effect of obesity on lung volumes. Thorax 2014; 69(8):752–9.
12. Khirfan G, Melillo CA, Al Abdi S, et al. Impact of esophageal pressure measurement on pulmonary hypertension diagnosis in patients with obesity. Chest 2022;162(3):684–92.
13. Sarma S, MacNamara JP, Balmain BN, et al. Challenging the hemodynamic hypothesis in heart failure with preserved ejection fraction: is exercise capacity limited by elevated pulmonary capillary wedge pressure? Circulation 2023;147(5):378–87.
14. Eisman AS, Shah RV, Dhakal BP, et al. Pulmonary capillary wedge pressure patterns during exercise predict exercise capacity and incident heart failure. Circ Heart Fail 2018;11(5):e004750.
15. Baratto C, Caravita S, Soranna D, et al. Current limitations of invasive exercise hemodynamics for the diagnosis of heart failure with preserved ejection fraction. Circ Heart Fail 2021;14(5):e007555.
16. Beard DA, Feigl EO. Understanding Guyton's venous return curves. Am J Physiol Heart Circ Physiol 2011;301(3):H629–33.
17. Trinity JD, Lee JF, Pahnke MD, et al. Attenuated relationship between cardiac output and oxygen uptake during high-intensity exercise. Acta Physiol 2012; 204(3):362–70.
18. Pandey A, Khera R, Park B, et al. Relative impairments in hemodynamic exercise reserve parameters in heart failure with preserved ejection fraction: a study-level pooled analysis. JACC Heart Fail 2018; 6(2):117–26.
19. Reddy YNV, Kaye DM, Handoko ML, et al. Diagnosis of heart failure with preserved ejection fraction among patients with unexplained dyspnea. JAMA Cardiol 2022;7(9):891–9.
20. Sarma S, MacNamara J, Livingston S, et al. Impact of severe obesity on exercise performance in heart failure with preserved ejection fraction. Physiol Rep 2020;8(22):e14634.
21. Bhella PS, Prasad A, Heinicke K, et al. Abnormal haemodynamic response to exercise in heart failure with preserved ejection fraction. Eur J Heart Fail 2011;13(12):1296–304.
22. Mascherbauer J, Zotter-Tufaro C, Duca F, et al. Wedge pressure rather than left ventricular end-diastolic pressure predicts outcome in heart failure with preserved ejection fraction. JACC Heart Fail 2017;5(11):795–801.
23. Shen MJ, Arora R, Jalife J. Atrial myopathy. JACC Basic Transl Sci 2019;4(5):640–54.
24. Reddy YNV, Obokata M, Verbrugge FH, et al. Atrial dysfunction in patients with heart failure with

preserved ejection fraction and atrial fibrillation. J Am Coll Cardiol 2020;76(9):1051–64.

25. Wolsk E, Bakkestrom R, Thomsen JH, et al. The influence of age on hemodynamic parameters during rest and exercise in healthy individuals. JACC Heart Fail 2017;5(5):337–46.

26. Oliveira RK, Agarwal M, Tracy JA, et al. Age-related upper limits of normal for maximum upright exercise pulmonary haemodynamics. Eur Respir J 2016; 47(4):1179–88.

27. Taivassalo T, Jensen TD, Kennaway N, et al. The spectrum of exercise tolerance in mitochondrial myopathies: a study of 40 patients. Brain 2003;126(Pt 2):413–23.

28. Astrand PO, Cuddy TE, Saltin B, et al. Cardiac output during submaximal and maximal work. J Appl Physiol 1964;19:268–74.

29. Julius S, Amery A, Whitlock LS, et al. Influence of age on the hemodynamic response to exercise. Circulation 1967;36(2):222–30.

30. Chomsky DB, Lang CC, Rayos GH, et al. Hemodynamic exercise testing. A valuable tool in the selection of cardiac transplantation candidates. Circulation 1996;94(12):3176–83.

31. Abudiab MM, Redfield MM, Melenovsky V, et al. Cardiac output response to exercise in relation to metabolic demand in heart failure with preserved ejection fraction. Eur J Heart Fail 2013;15(7): 776–85.

32. Dhakal BP, Malhotra R, Murphy RM, et al. Mechanisms of exercise intolerance in heart failure with preserved ejection fraction: the role of abnormal peripheral oxygen extraction. Circ Heart Fail 2015;8(2): 286–94.

33. Bevegard S, Holmgren A, Jonsson B. The effect of body position on the circulation at rest and during exercise, with special reference to the influence on the stroke volume. Acta Physiol Scand 1960;49: 279–98.

Cardiopulmonary Exercise Testing in Advanced Heart Failure Management

Isabela Landsteiner, MD[1], Takenori Ikoma, MD, PhD[1], Gregory D. Lewis, MD*

KEYWORDS

- Heart failure • Cardiac failure • Exercise testing • Cardiopulmonary exercise testing
- Disease management

KEY POINTS

- Patients with symptomatic heart failure with reduced ejection fraction exhibit marked functional impairment, evidenced by a mean peak VO_2 of 13.4 mL/kg/min (95% confidence interval [CI]: 12.2–14.6) in female individuals and 15.1 mL/kg/min (95% CI: 13.5–16.6) in male individuals.
- Cardiopulmonary exercise testing (CPET)-derived parameters, which extend beyond just peak VO_2, provide valuable information for accurate risk stratification in advanced heart failure.
- CPET permits comprehensive evaluation of multiorgan system deficits contributing to exercise intolerance, providing valuable information to guide clinical decisions related to advanced therapies in heart failure.

BACKGROUND

In the evaluation of advanced heart failure (HF), several cardiopulmonary exercise testing (CPET) parameters are employed to assess the physiologic limitations and prognostic outlook of patients. Each parameter provides distinct insights into the interplay among cardiovascular, respiratory, and peripheral systems under the stress of exercise. The subsequent sections offer a detailed examination of these key CPET parameters, emphasizing their clinical relevance and application in the management of advanced HF (**Table 1**).

APPROACH TO PERFORMING CARDIOPULMONARY EXERCISE TESTING IN PATIENTS WITH HEART FAILURE
Historical Context

Utilization of CPET among cardiologists caring for patients with HF has been historically underutilized. The need for specialized equipment (ie, a metabolic cart interfaced with a treadmill or cycle ergometer), the need to perform routine equipment calibration and troubleshooting, and the lack of standardized laboratory accreditation and staff competency assessment have posed challenges to widespread adoption of CPET. In addition, inadequate formal training of health professionals in CPET interpretation has curtailed widespread adoption of CPET among providers of cardiovascular care. Fortunately, modern metabolic carts that measure respiratory gas exchange during exercise have become smaller in size, easier to calibrate, and easier to interface with continuous electrocardiogram-monitoring, thereby facilitating establishment of CPET laboratories. Furthermore, modern metabolic cart software systems aid in gas exchange pattern recognition. Concomitantly, the physiologic and prognostic significance of gas exchange patterns has come into clearer focus through a growing

Cardiology Division and Cardiovascular Research Center, Massachusetts General Hospital, Boston, MA 02114, USA

[1] I. Landsteiner and T. Ikoma contributed equally.

* Corresponding author. Cardiology Division, Massachusetts General Hospital, Bigelow 800, 55 Fruit Street, Boston, MA 02114.
E-mail address: glewis@mgb.org

Heart Failure Clin 21 (2025) 35–49
https://doi.org/10.1016/j.hfc.2024.09.001
1551-7136/25/© 2024 Elsevier Inc. All rights reserved, including those for text and data mining, AI training, and similar technologies.

Table 1
Cardiopulmonary exercise testing and hemodynamic values for prognostic estimation in patients with advanced heart failure

CPET Variable	Intensity Level	Abnormal Threshold Value in HFrEF	Clinical Relevance	Calculation and Measurement Methods
Submaximal Oxygen Uptake Patterns				
MRT (s)	Initiation—low level	$\geq$60	Rate at which VO_2 increases to keep pace with the metabolic demands of initiating exercise. Delayed VO_2 augmentation is characteristic of HFrEF and incurs an "O_2 deficit" during exercise	Compare actual ΔVO_2 to idealized VO_2 if there was no delay in reaching steady state (O_2 deficit = time from rest to steady state $\times \Delta VO_2$ − cumulative, ΔVO_2)[13]
IW (W)	Initiation—low level	>25	Metabolic cost of initiating exercise, which is exaggerated in individuals with obesity	(Unloaded exercise VO_2 − rest VO_2)/(VO_2/WR)[4] to derive the workload equivalent of initiating exercise
Aerobic efficiency (mL/min/W)	During incremental ramp exercise	<8.5	Heightened reliance on anaerobic metabolism throughout exercise is characteristic of HFrEF, leading to a shallow slope <10 mL/min/W	$\Delta VO_2/\Delta WR$,[14] start the measurement 1 min after initiation of incremental ramp exercise
VO_2 at VAT (mL/kg/min)	Moderate	<9, <40% of predicted pVO_2	VO_2 at the ventilatory anaerobic metabolism	VO_2 value at VAT, identified from the inflection point of the VO_2 and VCO_2 slopes (V-slope method)[66]
OUES (L/min)	Throughout exercise	<1.47	Indicates VO_2 efficiency per unit of ventilation; higher values suggest better cardiopulmonary adaptation to exercise	Slope derived from plotting VO_2 against the logarithm of VE during incremental exercise[15]
Maximal Oxygen Uptake Patterns				
pVO_2 (mL/kg/min)	Peak	$\leq$14	The most reliable measure of cardiorespiratory fitness	Peak 30 s median VO_2 during the last minute of loaded exercise[5]

Parameter (units)	Timing	Value	Interpretation	Definition/formula
% Predicted pVO$_2$ (%)	Peak	<47%–50% predicted	Facilitates the comparison of pVO$_2$ between individuals of different age, sex, and body composition	Percentage of predicted pVO$_2$ based on gender, age, height, and weight (Wasserman and Hansen formula)[45]
O$_2$ pulse (mL/kg)	Peak	<85% of age-predicted value	Indicates the product of stroke volume and peripheral O$_2$ extraction	VO$_2$/HR[25] using the same approach as that used to derived pVO$_2$
Recovery Oxygen Uptake Patterns				
VO$_2$RD (s)	Recovery	>25	Indicates metabolic resilience following exercise	Time elapsed from the end of loaded exercise until VO$_2$ consistently drops below pVO$_2$[26]
Ventilatory Patterns				
VE/VCO$_2$ slope	Initiation—late	>36	Ventilatory efficiency	Slope of the VE and VCO$_2$ relationship[1]
EOV	Initiation	Observed	Cyclic oscillatory breathing during exercise	Cyclic ventilation fluctuations throughout for more than 60% of exercise, with an amplitude exceeding 15% of the resting average[67]
Ventilatory power (mm Hg)	Throughout exercise	≤3.5	Cardiovascular reserve in response to aerobic exercise	SBP$_{peak}$/(VE/VCO$_2$ slope)[33]
PETCO$_2$ (mm Hg)	Initiation	<36 at rest	Indicates ventilation/perfusion matching, but can be confounded by hyperventilation	End-tidal CO$_2$ in the resting state[52]
Hemodynamic Patterns (Noninvasive)				
SBP (mm Hg)	Peak	<120	Indicates impaired cardiac reserve function	SBP at the end of incremental exercise[53]
Circulatory power (mm Hg·mL/min/kg)	Throughout exercise	≤1750	Surrogate of cardiac power, providing information on cardiac systolic function	VO$_2$ peak × SBP$_{peak}$[33,34]
PrPP (mm Hg)	Throughout exercise	0.48	Indicates left ventricular contractile reserve function	(SBP − DBP)/SBP[36]

(continued on next page)

Table 1
(continued)

CPET Variable	Intensity Level	Abnormal Threshold Value in HFrEF	Clinical Relevance	Calculation and Measurement Methods
HR recovery (bpm)	Recovery	≤6 at 1 min	Indicates autonomic system function	(HR 1 min after peak exercise) − (HR at peak exercise)[37]
Hemodynamic gain index (bpm/mm Hg)	Rest and peak	<1.1 (Men) <1.27 (Women)	Evaluate hemodynamic changes using HR and SBP	$(HR_{peak} \times SBP_{peak} - HR_{rest} \times SBP_{rest}) / (HR_{rest} \times SBP_{rest})$[55,56]
Hemodynamic Patterns (Invasive)				
PCWP/CO slope (mm Hg/L/min)	Throughout exercise	>2	Integrated measure of left heart filling pressure and cardiac performance	Slope of the relationship between PCWP and CO from rest to peak exercise[61]
Cardiac power (W)	Peak	<2	Measure of cardiac function integrating flow generated by the heart and peripheral perfusion pressure	(mean arterial pressure − RAP) × CO × 222.10^{-5} [42]
CavO₂ (mL/dL)	Peak	≤14	Peripheral oxygen extraction, low values invoke extracardiac limitations to exercise performance	Arterial-mixed venous O₂ content difference[47]

Abbreviations: CavO₂, arterial-mixed venous oxygen content difference; CO, cardiac output; CO₂, carbon dioxide; CPET, cardiopulmonary exercise testing; CV, cardiovascular; DBP, diastolic blood pressure; EOV, exercise oscillatory ventilation; HF, heart failure; HFrEF, heart failure with reduced ejection fraction; HR, heart rate; IW, internal work; MRT, mean response time; O₂, oxygen; OUES, O₂ uptake efficiency slope; PCWP, pulmonary capillary wedge pressure; PETCO₂, end-tidal CO₂; PrPP, proportionate pulse pressure; pVO₂, peak oxygen uptake; RAP, right atrial pressure; SBP, systolic blood pressure; SV, systolic volume; VAT, ventilatory anaerobic threshold; VE, ventilation; VE/VCO₂, ratio of minute ventilation to carbon dioxide production; VO₂, oxygen uptake; VO₂RD, VO₂ recovery delay; WR, work rate.

body of research in applied CPET that has been endorsed by scientific statements.[1–3]

Pretest Evaluation

Prior to conducting a CPET, it is important to perform a careful patient evaluation. Patients should be specifically asked about conditions that preclude incremental ramp exercise (**Fig. 1**). It is particularly important to ascertain transient extracardiac conditions that impair exercise tolerance or if a patient is experiencing acute HF exacerbation, either of which should trigger the decision to defer CPET until these issues are resolved or optimized such the CPET findings are representative of usual health status. Similarly, usual medications should be continued to ensure exercise is conducted in the setting of exposure to clinically indicated medications. Additionally, for those with implantable electrical devices, it is important to confirm device settings, particularly the heart rate (HR) trigger for antitachycardia therapies, to ensure this threshold is not reached during maximum incremental ramp exercise.

Cardiopulmonary Exercise Testing Protocol Implementation

A 3 to 5 minute period of resting gas exchange measurement permits patients to become accustomed to breathing into the mouthpiece or face mask without hyperventilation. Hyperventilation can confound subsequent exercise gas exchange measurements. A low initial work rate is critical to avoid rapid cessation of exercise in patients with severe HF. We recommend an initial 3 minute period of unloaded exercise (0 W, or the lowest workload setting permissible on a cycle ergometer, or walking on a treadmill with no incline at <1.8 miles per hour [mph]) in order to quantify the isolated metabolic cost of moving the legs (ie, internal work [IW])[4] prior to the measurement of oxygen uptake (VO_2)–work rate relationships during incremental ramp exercise (ie, external work). Because the linearity of O_2 uptake during early exercise is used to ascertain the ventilatory anaerobic threshold (VAT),[5] it is important to be confident of the linearity of the work rate profile that yielded the response.[6] For cycle ergometry, approximately 10 W/min increment is usually appropriate based on previous studies in HF demonstrating achieved workloads of 50 to 90 W, which translates to the desired duration of testing (8–12 minutes) shown to optimize peak VO_2 (pVO_2) measurement.[7] Treadmill protocols should also consist of a gradual increment in speed and grade with approximately 10 W/min ramp (for a 70 kg individual), which is the case for the modified Naughton Protocol used in the Heart Failure: A

Controlled Trial Investigating Outcomes of Exercise Training (HF-ACTION) trial[8] and a customized HF protocol currently used in the HF studies supported by the Massachusetts General Hospital CPET Core Laboratory.[9] Of note, treadmill testing, compared to cycle ergometry, results in 7% to 11% higher pVO_2 values because of the activation of more muscle mass with treadmill exercise.[10]

The patient-limited nature of maximum exercise with CPET, coupled with an individualized gradual incremental ramp (5–25 W/min), makes the procedure feasible and safe even in patients with advanced HF. In a study of greater than 9000 CPETs, the adverse event rates ranged from 0.045% to 0.16% (primarily ventricular tachyarrhythmias), and there were no deaths in the investigation of over 9000 CPETs performed in populations enriched for HF.[11,12]

PHYSIOLOGIC BASIS FOR SPECIFIC CARDIOPULMONARY EXERCISE TESTING PARAMETERS AND APPROACH TO THEIR MEASUREMENTS
Submaximal Oxygen Uptake Patterns

While pVO_2 often serves as a focal point of CPET reporting, it is important to recognize that CPET captures oxygen uptake patterns starting at rest and throughout incremental exercise. At rest, expected VO_2 is 3.5 mL/kg/min or 1 metabolic equivalent. In a recent large community-based CPET study, we found that average measured resting VO_2 was 3.50 mL/kg/min, suggesting that resting CPET can accurately capture resting gas exchange measures. Upon initiation of exercise, the *mean response time* (MRT) refers to the average time required for VO_2 to reach a steady state during low-level exercise. It represents the time constant of the exponential rise in VO_2, indicating how swiftly the body can respond to the increased O_2 delivery demands of skeletal muscles during exercise. In patients with HF with reduced ejection fraction (HFrEF), an MRT greater than 60 seconds was closely related to reduced exercise Fick cardiac output (CO) and elevated biventricular filling pressures.[13]

Internal work

IW is a body mass index (BMI)-related measure that quantifies the work equivalents required to initiate unloaded exercise and reflects the metabolic cost of initiating movement. High IW with expenditure of "VO_2 reserve" leads to less capacity to perform "external work." Significant between-patient heterogeneity in IW means that a given task, such as climbing a flight of stairs, comes as markedly different "metabolic costs" as measured by absolute values of VO_2.[4] While

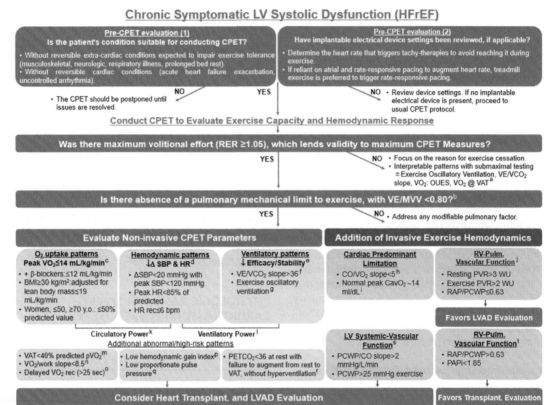

Fig. 1. Flowchart of evaluation and patient selection for advanced heart failure intervention. [a]OUES of less than 1.47 and VO_2 at VAT less than 9 mL/kg/min indicate a poor prognosis.[15,46] [b]VE/MVV ≥ 0.80 indicates low breathing reserve.[47] [c]Peak VO_2 values must be interpreted in the context of the patient's age, sex, size, and background.[49] [d]Lack of SBP augmentation, chronotropic incompetence, and slow HR recovery are associated with poor prognosis.[37,53,54] [e]Ventilatory inefficiency and oscillation during exercise are related with poor outcome.[30] [f]Identifies high-risk patients and offers prognostic insights beyond peak VO_2 (Wasserman K. NY: Futura Pub. Co. 2002).[1] [g]Presence of EOV is reliably linked to a 1 year mortality rate exceeding 20%.[30,51] [h]Degree of disparity between the rise in systemic O_2 delivery and the corresponding increase in oxygen consumption.[68,69] [i]Indicative of peripheral O_2 extraction.[47] [j]In patients with pulmonary hypertension, LVAD is preferred initially, instead of transplantation to lower PVR.[49] [k]Calculated from peak $VO_2 \times SBP_{peak}$. Low circulatory power is associated with worse outcomes compared to those with low peak VO_2 but preserved circulatory power.[70] [l]Ratio of SBP_{peak} to the VE/VCO$_2$ slope, with a lower value indicating a severely impaired cardiovascular reserve in response to exercise.[33,71] [m]Low VAT predicts early mortality.[72] [n]Low VO_2/work suggests inefficient aerobic work.[14] [o]Duration from the end of incremental exercise until VO_2 permanently falls below peak VO_2. Delayed VO_2 recovery time indicates impaired cardiac output augmentation during exercise and is linked to poor outcomes.[26] [p] HGI: Integrated marker of hemodynamic reserve calculated from the equation of $(HR_{peak} \times SBP_{peak} - HR_{rest} \times SBP_{rest})/(HR_{rest} \times SBP_{rest})$. HGI less than 1.1 for men and HGI less than 1.27 for women indicate poor prognosis.[55,56] [q]PrPP: Ratio of pulse pressure to SBP. Lower exercise PrPP is associated with higher risk of adverse cardiovascular outcomes.[36] [r]Decreased PETCO$_2$ indicates deficits in functional, ventilatory, and cardiac performance during exercise.[52] PETCO$_2$ is expected to rise by 3 to 6 mm Hg from rest to VAT. [s]Captures the change in cardiac output relative to increases in left heart filling pressure during exercise, predicts outcomes.[20,21] [t]Indicates biventricular dysfunction, suggesting direct transplantation instead of LVAD.[49] CavO$_2$, arterial-mixed venous oxygen content difference; BMI, body mass index; CO, cardiac output; CPET, cardiopulmonary exercise testing; HFrEF, heart failure with reduced ejection fraction; HR, heart rate; LVAD, left ventricular assist device; LV, left ventricle; MVV, maximal voluntary ventilation; OUES, oxygen uptake efficiency slope; PAPi, pulmonary artery pulsatility index; PCWP, pulmonary capillary wedge pressure; PET, partial pressure of end-tidal; Pulm., pulmonary; PVR, pulmonary vascular resistance; RAP, right atrium pressure; rec, recovery; rec, recovery; RER, respiratory exchange ratio; RV, right ventricle; SBP, systolic blood pressure; VAT, ventilatory anaerobic threshold; VE, minute ventilation; VE/VCO$_2$, ratio of minute ventilation to carbon dioxide production; VO_2, oxygen uptake.

the period of unloaded exercise is utilized to derive MRT and IW, once the incremental ramp portion of exercise is initiated it permits assessment of the VO_2/work slope, termed *aerobic efficiency*.

Aerobic efficiency

Represents the slope of oxygen utilization to the amount of work performed with normal values around 10 ± 1.5 mL/min/W.[14] Individuals with higher aerobic efficiency tend to exhibit a steeper VO_2-work rate slope, indicating greater reliance on aerobic metabolism and higher pVO_2 values. Conversely, lower VO_2-work rate slopes suggest reduced efficiency, often seen in patients with HF, where there is a greater dependence on anaerobic metabolism to perform work during exercise.

Ventilatory anaerobic threshold

During increasing workload exercise, energy production shifts from an aerobic metabolism to a state combining aerobic and anaerobic metabolism. Throughout the initial aerobic phase of the exercise, which lasts until about 50% to 60% of pVO_2 is achieved, CO_2 elimination (VCO_2) increases linearly with VO_2. In the latter half of exercise, there is a transition toward an anaerobic metabolism. The VAT, usually determined by visual assessment (the V-slope method), represents this specific point at which VCO_2 starts to rise exponentially relative to VO_2 due to the onset of anaerobic metabolism with buffering of lactate responsible for excess CO_2 production relative to O_2 uptake.

O_2 uptake efficiency slope

O_2 uptake efficiency slope (OUES) is the index between VO_2 and the logarithm of (VE) throughout the exercise. OUES differs less than 2% when derived from 75%, 90%, or 100% of exercise duration. OUES represents an objective and reproducible measure of cardiopulmonary reserve that can be derived from submaximal exercise effort.[15]

Maximal Exercise Oxygen Uptake Patterns

Peak VO_2

pVO_2 is the highest value of VO_2 obtained during maximal symptom-limited CPET and is considered the gold standard method to assess functional capacity. It reflects the integrative capacity of the cardiovascular, respiratory, and peripheral systems to transport and utilize oxygen during maximal exercise. It is directly related to components of the Fick equation at peak exercise:[2,16]

Taking into account 6 studies reporting sex-specific pVO_2 among 14,313 patients with symptomatic HFrEF,[17–22] we found that female individuals achieved a mean pVO_2 of 13.4 mL/kg/min (95% confidence interval [CI]: 12.2 to 14.6), and male

individuals achieved a mean pVO_2 of 15.1 mL/kg/min (95% CI: 13.5–16.6; **Fig. 2**), highlighting significant exercise capacity limitations in both groups. Female patients with HFrEF showed a pVO_2 1.7 (95% CI: 1.3–2.0) mL/kg/min lower than male patients, which reflects lower stroke volume in the setting of the smaller left ventricular chamber sizes and less lean mass.[23,24]

Considering the metabolic cost of activities relative to pVO_2 achieved by patients with symptomatic HFrEF, significant functional limitations are evident (see **Fig. 2**). For example, walking at 3 mph comes at a metabolic cost that is more than 66% of the maximum "metabolic cost" the average symptomatic patient with HFrEF can afford. More vigorous activities, such as jogging 5 mph, are well-beyond the average pVO_2s that patients with HFrEF can afford. Furthermore, engaging in more strenuous activities, such as jogging 5 mph, is not feasible for many patients with HFrEF.

Oxygen pulse

Oxygen pulse (O_2 pulse) is the ratio of VO_2 and HR, which is equal to the product of stroke volume and arterial-to-mixed venous O_2 content ($CavO_2$). O_2 pulse reflects both cardiac performance coupled and peripheral O_2 extraction, but does not distinguish between relative abnormalities in these 2 variables that compose O_2 pulse.[25]

Postexercise Recovery Oxygen Uptake Patterns

VO_2 recovery delay

VO_2 recovery delay (VO_2RD) is a metric of the duration of time from the end of loaded exercise until VO_2 permanently falls below pVO_2 (**Fig. 3**A). VO_2RD can also be expressed as $T_{1/2}$, which represents the time for VO_2 to decrease to 50% of pVO_2 adjusted for individual resting VO_2.[26] VO_2RD highlights the dynamics of how quickly VO_2 returns to baseline, providing insights into the body's ability to restore metabolic homeostasis after exertion. In healthy subjects, VO_2 declines almost immediately after peak exercise, whereas in patients with HF, VO_2RD is consistently prolonged.[26–28] This prolonged VO_2RD has been associated with poorer cardiac performance during exercise and an increased risk of adverse outcomes in HF (**Fig. 3**B).[26,27]

Ventilatory Patterns

Minute ventilation/carbon dioxide elimination slope

The VE/VCO_2 slope is the ratio between minute ventilation (VE) and VCO_2, and it measures the amount of VE required to eliminate 1 L of CO_2.[16]

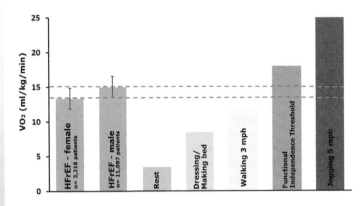

Fig. 2. Metabolic cost of activities relative to peak VO_2 in symptomatic heart failure with reduced ejection fraction stratified by sex. HFrEF; heart failure with reduced ejection fraction.

It indicates the state of ventilatory efficiency and is composed of 2 variables, fractional dead space relative to tidal volume, which reflects the adequacy with which the right heart supports ventilation-perfusion matching, and $PaCO_2$ for which lower set points are characteristic of HFrEF and pulmonary arterial hypertension. In patients with HFrEF, the VE/VCO_2 slope was directly related to pulmonary vascular resistance (PVR) and indirectly correlated to right ventricular ejection fraction during exercise.[29] Furthermore, changes in VE/VCO_2 slope in response to phosphodiesterase 5 inhibition in patients with HFrEF and elevated PVR occurred proportionately to changes in exercise PVR and right ventricular ejection fraction. Assessment of VE/VCO_2 in advanced HF has a significant role since alteration in pulmonary vasomotor tone during exercise has a major role in determining ventilatory efficiency in these patients.[29]

Exercise oscillatory ventilation

Exercise oscillatory ventilation (EOV) is an abnormal breathing pattern observed during exercise, characterized by regular cyclic fluctuations in VE with a typical cycle length of around 1 minute. While prevalence varies across studies, it is more common within cohorts with advanced HF.[30,31] Mechanisms driving EOV may include reduced CO leading to circulatory delay, increased chemosensitivity to blood gases, and impaired autonomic regulation, all of which contribute to the instability of the ventilatory control system during exercise.[32]

Ventilatory power

Ventilatory power is defined as the ratio of peak systolic blood pressure (BP) to VE/VCO_2 slope. It serves as a composite measure that reflects both ventilatory efficiency and cardiovascular performance.[33]

Hemodynamics Patterns

Circulatory power

Circulatory power, defined as the product of pVO_2 and peak systolic blood pressure (SBP), is a valuable surrogate for cardiac power, providing significant information on cardiac systolic function.[34] In a cohort of 219 patients with chronic HR, circulatory power was found to have a direct relation with cardiac power with an overall Pearson's correlation of 0.84 at peak exercise ($P<.0001$).[35]

Proportionate pulse pressure

Proportionate pulse pressure (PrPP) is the ratio of pulse pressure to SBP, with pulse pressure defined as systolic minus diastolic BP. In patients with HFrEF, higher PrPP is associated with preserved left ventricular contractile reserve. In a study by Namasivayam and colleagues,[36] HFrEF patients with lower exercise PrPP were shown to have lower peak exercise stroke volume ($P = .013$).

Heart rate recovery

Heart rate recovery (HRR) is defined as the reduction in HR measured 1 or 2 minutes after the cessation of exercise. A prolonged HRR, characterized by a slower decline in HR, has been associated with autonomic dysfunction and is considered an indicator of impaired parasympathetic reactivation.[37]

INVASIVE EXERCISE HEMODYNAMICS IN ADVANCED HEART FAILURE

Invasive CPET has several advantages over noninvasive exercise testing, being regarded as the gold standard assessment for exertional dyspnea.[38,39] Invasive CPET has the distinct ability to determine the relative contributions of each underlying condition to a patient's symptoms.[40] In patients with HF undergoing evaluation for advanced therapies,

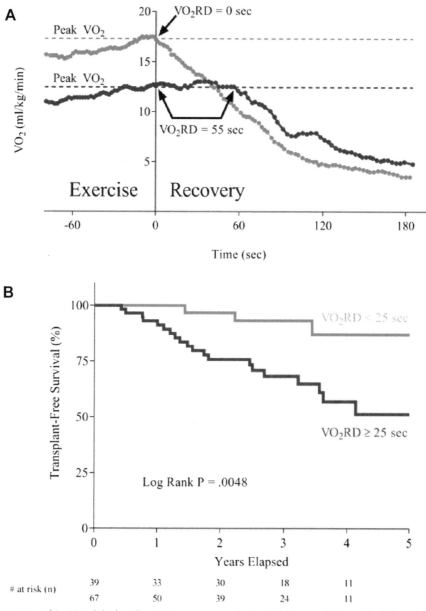

Fig. 3. VO$_2$ recovery kinetics. (*A*) This illustration compares 2 heart failure patients with different VO$_2$ recovery delay (VO$_2$RD) patterns. The gray area represents the final phase of incremental ramp exercise. VO$_2$RD is defined as the time from the end of exercise until VO$_2$ permanently drops below peak VO$_2$ (*dashed lines*). The blue line shows a patient whose VO$_2$ immediately decreases after exercise, resulting in a VO$_2$RD of 0 seconds. The red line represents a patient whose VO$_2$ remains at or above peak levels for 55 seconds postexercise before beginning to decline. (*B*) Kaplan–Meier transplant-free survival curves for HFrEF (n = 106 patients) dichotomized by VO$_2$RD of 25 seconds, highlighting VO$_2$RD as a prognostic indicator in HFrEF. HFrEF, heart failure with reduced ejection fraction; VO$_2$RD, VO$_2$ recovery delay. (Figure reproduced from Bailey et al.: Post-Exercise Oxygen Uptake Recovery Delay: A Novel Index of Impaired Cardiac Reserve Capacity in Heart Failure.[26])

invasive CPET helps determine the extent to which exercise limitation is related to cardiac function, allowing for the identification of cardiocentric limitations while also assessing for peripheral factors beyond the heart.

Invasive CPET enables the simultaneous measurement of VO$_2$ and CavO$_2$, allowing for the calculation of minute-by-minute Fick COs. Additionally, it provides detailed assessments of right atrial pressure (RAP), pulmonary arterial pressure

(PAP), and pulmonary capillary wedge pressure (PCWP), which together help to accurately define the pressure–flow relationships within the cardiovascular system. In comparison to single-unit measurements during peak exercise, the slopes derived from multiple data points of pressures and CO throughout exercise provide the advantage of reducing the influence of peak exercise respirophasic pressure swings.[41]

Cardiac Power

Cardiac power is a key indicator of the heart's pumping efficiency, derived from the principles of fluid dynamics, where power equals the product of pressure and flow. Specifically, cardiac power is calculated as the product of CO and mean arterial pressure, integrating both blood flow generated by the heart and peripheral perfusion pressure. This makes cardiac power a comprehensive measure of cardiac function, capturing the interplay between flow and pressure within the cardiovascular system.[42]

SAFETY OF CARDIOPULMONARY EXERCISE TESTING

Incremental ramp CPET has been shown to be a very safe procedure, even in patients with high-risk cardiac diseases. In a single retrospective review on the safety of CPET, Skalski and colleagues[11] examined results from 5060 tests from 4250 high-risk patients, including conditions such as HF, hypertrophic cardiomyopathy, known coronary artery disease (CAD), valvular heart disease, prior cardiac transplantation, and history of cardiac arrest. Despite the high-risk features of the studied population, there were no fatal events, and only 8 adverse events occurred (0.16% event rate), which was more commonly related to sustained ventricular tachycardia in 6 cases, which all self-terminated without intervention. There was one myocardial infarction in a postheart transplant patient, and another patient with known CAD developed severe dyspnea.[11]

A study by Keteyian and colleagues[12] evaluated 4411 CPETs from 2331 patients with HFrEF and left ventricular ejection fraction (LVEF) 35% or less who were enrolled in the prospective HF-ACTION trial. There were no deaths, exacerbation of HF requiring hospitalization, myocardial infarctions, strokes, or transient ischemic attacks. There was 1 episode of ventricular fibrillation and 1 episode of supraventricular tachycardia, resulting in 0.45 nonfatal major cardiovascular events per 1000 exercise tests.[12]

RISK STRATIFICATION AND PATIENT SELECTION FOR ADVANCED HEART FAILURE INTERVENTIONS

Managing patients with HF is inherently complex.[43] Providing precise prognostic information is essential, particularly for patients with severe HF who are at high risk of mortality. This allows both patients and health care providers to make informed decisions regarding advanced therapeutic options, such as left ventricular assist device (LVAD) implantation and heart transplantation. While these interventions carry inherent procedural risks, these treatments also offer the potential to significantly improve the quality of life and overall prognosis for patients with HF with cardiocentric limitations to exercise performance.

CPET is essential in the selection of candidates for heart transplantation and LVAD implantation in advanced HF. While it is generally conducted safely in patients with cardiovascular diseases,[44] pre-CPET evaluation is crucial (see **Fig. 1**). The initial step in CPET evaluation is to determine whether the patient exerted maximal volitional effort, typically identified by a respiratory exchange ratio (RER) of 1.05 or greater.[45] If the patient does not achieve an RER of 1.05 or higher, the reason for exercise cessation should be investigated. In those cases, attention should be directed toward oxygen uptake variables that do not rely on maximum voluntary effort. An OUES below 1.47 and reduced VO_2 at VAT are examples of variables derived during submaximum exercise that predict suggest a poor prognosis.[15,16,46] If the patient exhibits a ratio of VE to maximal voluntary ventilation (MVV) greater than 80%, a pulmonary mechanical limitation is suspected.[47]

Among O_2 uptake patterns, pVO_2 remains the primary fitness metric and should be the central focus of CPET interpretation for prognostication. The landmark study by Mancini and colleagues[48] established pVO_2 of 14 mL/kg/min or less as a critical threshold, indicating a poor prognosis and serving as a key criterion for heart transplantation candidacy. Specifically, the study identified pVO_2 of 14 mL/kg/min or less as a criterion for which 1 year survival was lower than the survival achieved through transplantation, suggesting that symptomatic HF patients with pVO_2 greater than 14 mL/kg/min may be safely deferred from cardiac transplantation.[48] For specific patient populations, other thresholds should be applied: a more conservative threshold of 12 mL/kg/min or less is recommended for patients on beta-blockers, pVO_2 adjusted for lean body mass of 19 mL/kg/min or less for patients with obesity

(BMI ≥ 30 kg/m^2), and for women or patients aged 50 years or less or subjects aged 70 years or older, pVO$_2$ should be evaluated as a percentage of the predicted value, with levels below approximately 50% indicating a poor prognosis.[49]

In terms of ventilatory efficiency and stability, a VE/VCO$_2$ slope greater than 36 is correlated with high-risk HF and predicts a worse prognosis in keeping with the recognized critical role of right heart and pulmonary vascular function in predicting prognosis in HFrEF.[1] A recent study by Nadruz and colleagues[50] demonstrated that both pVO$_2$ and VE/VCO$_2$ values effectively predict prognosis of patients with HF, irrespective of LVEF (**Fig. 4**).

The presence of EOV is among the strongest indicators of adverse outcomes in HF with its presence being linked to a 1 year mortality rate exceeding 20%.[14,51] In addition, ventilatory power has been shown to be a strong and independent predictor of cardiac events in patients with HF,[33] and a low partial pressure of end-tidal CO$_2$ (PETCO$_2$) is associated with poor augmentation disorder and indicates ventilatory pattern impairment.[52]

In the assessment of hemodynamic patterns, the inability to reach an SBP of 120 mm Hg or greater and a failure to increase SBP during exercise to 20 mm Hg or greater are associated with a poor prognosis, particularly when combined with a pVO$_2$ of 14 mL/kg/min or less or diminished CO augmentation.[53,54] A study by Cohen-Solal and colleagues,[34] including 175 patients with chronic HFrEF, revealed that circulatory power was a strong predictor of outcomes, especially in the subgroup of patients with low pVO$_2$ and peak BP. HFrEF patients with low exercise PrPP were also shown to have a higher risk of adverse cardiovascular events.[36] A low hemodynamic gain index is associated with the hemodynamic pattern,[36,55,56] and a slow HR recovery of 6 or less beats per minute predicts poor outcomes.[37]

MULTIVARIATE CARDIOPULMONARY EXERCISE TESTING RISK-ASSESSMENT APPROACHES

The ability to combine multiple CPET variables for risk stratification is inherently attractive and starts to address the issue of how to interpret potentially discordant CPET patterns as they relate to risk stratification. The Metabolic Exercise Cardiac Kidney Index (MECKI) score incorporates pVO$_2$ and VE/VCO$_2$ slope to predict the likelihood of LVAD implantation and HF-related mortality within 2 years.[57] Additionally, a prognostic approach combining pVO$_2$, VE/VCO$_2$ slope, and the presence of EOV,

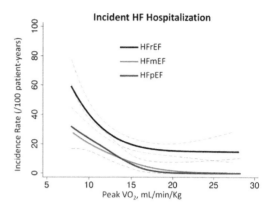

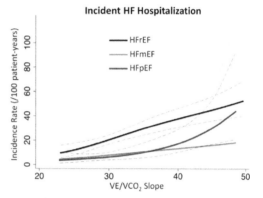

Fig. 4. Adjusted incidence rates of HF hospitalizations by peak VO$_2$ and VE/VCO$_2$ slope across HFrEF, HFmEF, and HFpEF groups. HF, heart failure; HFmEF, heart failure with mildly reduced ejection fraction; HFpEF, heart failure with preserved ejection fraction; HFrEF, heart failure with reduced ejection fraction. (Nadruz, W. et al., (2017). Prognostic value of cardiopulmonary exercise testing in heart failure with reduced, mid-range, and preserved ejection fraction. Journal of the American Heart Association, 6(11). https://doi.org/10.1161/jaha.117.006000.)

reflecting impaired hemodynamic response to exercise, has also been described.[16,32]

Additionally, Lala and colleagues[58] analyzed CPET data from the Registry Evaluation of Vital Information for VADs in Ambulatory Life (REVIVAL), which included patients with advanced HF, and found that VE/VCO$_2$ slope and circulatory power were effective in predicting adverse outcomes.

INVASIVE HEMODYNAMIC MEASUREMENTS DURING EXERCISE IN HEART FAILURE WITH REDUCED EJECTION FRACTION

Parameters provided by invasive exercise hemodynamics are also valuable. In a study by Chomsky and colleagues,[59] including 185 ambulatory patients with HF referred for cardiac transplantation, exercise CO response was the strongest independent predictor of survival according to both univariate and multivariate analyses. The overall 1 year survival rate was 72% for patients with reduced CO response and 38% for those with reduced CO response and pVO_2 of 10 mL/min/kg or less. Peak cardiac power output has also been shown to be an independent predictor of outcome.[42,60]

Our group has described a steep PCWP/CO slope during exercise in both HFrEF and heart failure with preserved ejection fraction (HFpEF), with values greater than 2 mm Hg/L/min was associated with adverse cardiac outcomes.[61] Additionally, in patients with chronic exertional dyspnea, a PAP/CO slope greater than 3 mm Hg/L/min was associated with a 2 fold increase in the hazard of future cardiovascular or death events.[62] A shallow CO/VO_2 slope is indicative of a predominant cardiac limitation during exercise.[47,63]

For patients with irreversible precapillary pulmonary hypertension, with high resting PVR and an inadequate response to the acute vasodilator challenge, LVAD implantation should be considered instead of heart transplantation, in order to lower PVR. Repeated measures of PAP and PCWP during exercise provides heightened hemodynamic resolution in parsing relative burdens of precapillary and postcapillary pulmonary hypertension, which can aid in deciding whether a patient should be supported with an LVAD to lower PVR versus proceeding directly to heart transplantation.

CARDIOPULMONARY EXERCISE TESTING ASSESSMENT IN ADVANCED MECHANICAL SUPPORT THERAPY

CPET is also useful for the evaluation after LVAD implantation. It is recommended as an objective assessment of functional capacity[49] and can be informative in decision-making regarding LVAD explanation. Proposed CPET criterion for explant consideration is either pVO_2 greater than 16 mL/kg/min or a VE/VCO_2 slope less than 34 during low LVAD speed testing.[64] However, direct assessments of cardiac performance with invasive exercise hemodynamics are desirable in considering LVAD explantation, particularly the PCWP/CO slope, and assessment of peripheral oxygen extraction, which may be quite variable among patients.[65]

SUMMARY

CPET informs the management of advanced HF, providing comprehensive insights into the multiorgan reserve capacity, risk stratification, and patient-specific therapeutic decision-making.

CPET-derived parameters enable clinicians to more accurately assess risk, guide the selection of candidates for advanced therapies such as heart transplantation and LVAD implantation, and monitor postintervention functional capacity. Additionally, the integration of CPET with invasive exercise hemodynamics allows for a thorough evaluation of the relative cardiac and extracardiac deficits in exercise tolerance. As the therapeutic landscape continues to evolve, CPET remains an essential tool for optimizing patient care, providing objective data that support personalized and evidence-based clinical decision-making.

CLINICS CARE POINTS

- Patients with advanced HF should be considered for CPET to guide clinical decision-making for advanced therapies.

- A maximal CPET should be performed after a pre-CPET evaluation that includes assessing the patient's suitability and reviewing implantable electrical device settings.

- A maximal CPET is considered when the RER is 1.05 or greater. In the case of a submaximal CPET, the interpretation should be focused on submaximal patterns.

- When a maximal CPET is achieved, a pVO_2 cutoff point for advanced HF therapies is 14 mL/kg/min or less if not on beta-blocker, 12 mL/kg/min or less if on beta-blocker, and less than 50% of predicted values for women or extreme age patients.

- The addition of invasive exercise hemodynamics offers valuable information on the right ventricular-pulmonary vascular reserve and variable peripheral contributions to exercise intolerance and helps to guide decision-making for appropriateness of advanced HF interventions.

DISCLOSURE

The authors have nothing to disclose.

FUNDING

Funder: Heart Failure Research Innovation Fund.

REFERENCES

1. Arena R, Myers J, Abella J, et al. Development of a ventilatory classification system in patients with heart failure. Circulation 2007;115(18):2410–7.

2. Balady GJ, Arena R, Sietsema K, et al. Clinician's Guide to cardiopulmonary exercise testing in adults: a scientific statement from the American Heart Association. Circulation 2010;122(2):191–225.

3. Gibbons RJ, Araoz PA, Williamson EE. The year in cardiac imaging. J Am Coll Cardiol 2010;55(5):483–95.

4. Shah RV, Schoenike MW, Armengol de la Hoz M, et al. Metabolic cost of exercise initiation in patients with heart failure with preserved ejection fraction vs community-dwelling adults. JAMA Cardiol 2021;6(6):653–60.

5. Sue DY, Wasserman K, Moricca RB, et al. Metabolic acidosis during exercise in patients with chronic obstructive pulmonary disease. Use of the V-slope method for anaerobic threshold determination. Chest 1988;94(5):931–8.

6. ATS/ACCP Statement on cardiopulmonary exercise testing. Am J Respir Crit Care Med 2003;167(2):211–77.

7. Buchfuhrer MJ, Hansen JE, Robinson TE, et al. Optimizing the exercise protocol for cardiopulmonary assessment. J Appl Physiol Respir Environ Exerc Physiol 1983;55(5):1558–64.

8. O'Connor CM, Whellan DJ, Lee KL, et al. Efficacy and safety of exercise training in patients with chronic heart failure: HF-ACTION randomized controlled trial. JAMA 2009;301(14):1439–50.

9. Lewis GD, Docherty KF, Voors AA, et al. Developments in exercise capacity assessment in heart failure clinical trials and the rationale for the design of METEORIC-HF. Circ Heart Fail 2022;15(5):e008970.

10. Shephard RJ. Tests of maximum oxygen intake. A critical review. Sports Med 1984;1(2):99–124.

11. Skalski J, Allison TG, Miller TD. The safety of cardiopulmonary exercise testing in a population with high-risk cardiovascular diseases. Circulation 2012;126(21):2465–72.

12. Keteyian SJ, Isaac D, Thadani U, et al. Safety of symptom-limited cardiopulmonary exercise testing in patients with chronic heart failure due to severe left ventricular systolic dysfunction. Am Heart J 2009;158(4 Suppl):S72–7.

13. Chatterjee NA, Murphy RM, Malhotra R, et al. Prolonged mean VO2 response time in systolic heart failure: an indicator of impaired right ventricular-pulmonary vascular function. Circ Heart Fail 2013;6(3):499–507.

14. Tanabe Y, Nakagawa I, Ito E, et al. Hemodynamic basis of the reduced oxygen uptake relative to work rate during incremental exercise in patients with chronic heart failure. Int J Cardiol 2002;83(1):57–62.

15. Hollenberg M, Tager IB. Oxygen uptake efficiency slope: an index of exercise performance and cardiopulmonary reserve requiring only submaximal exercise. J Am Coll Cardiol 2000;36(1):194–201.

16. Malhotra R, Bakken K, D'Elia E, et al. Cardiopulmonary exercise testing in heart failure. JACC Heart failure 2016;4(8):607–16.

17. Keteyian SJ, Patel M, Kraus WE, et al. Variables measured during cardiopulmonary exercise testing as predictors of mortality in chronic systolic heart failure. J Am Coll Cardiol 2016;67(7):780–9.

18. Brawner CA, Shafiq A, Aldred HA, et al. Comprehensive analysis of cardiopulmonary exercise testing and mortality in patients with systolic heart failure: the Henry Ford Hospital cardiopulmonary exercise testing (FIT-CPX) project. J Card Fail 2015;21(9):710–8.

19. Grilli G, Salvioni E, Moscucci F, et al. A matter of sex-persistent predictive value of MECKI score prognostic power in men and women with heart failure and reduced ejection fraction: a multicenter study. Frontiers in cardiovascular medicine 2024;11:1390544.

20. Corrà U, Mezzani A, Giordano A, et al. Peak oxygen consumption and prognosis in heart failure: 14 mL/kg/min is not a "gender-neutral" reference. Int J Cardiol 2013;167(1):157–61.

21. Elmariah S, Goldberg LR, Allen MT, et al. Effects of gender on peak oxygen consumption and the timing of cardiac transplantation. J Am Coll Cardiol 2006;47(11):2237–42.

22. Hsich E, Chadalavada S, Krishnaswamy G, et al. Long-term prognostic value of peak oxygen consumption in women versus men with heart failure and severely impaired left ventricular systolic function. Am J Cardiol 2007;100(2):291–5.

23. Beale AL, Meyer P, Marwick TH, et al. Sex differences in cardiovascular pathophysiology: why women are overrepresented in heart failure with preserved ejection fraction. Circulation 2018;138(2):198–205.

24. Karastergiou K, Smith SR, Greenberg AS, et al. Sex differences in human adipose tissues - the biology of pear shape. Biol Sex Differ 2012;3(1):13.

25. Oliveira RB, Myers J, Araújo CG, et al. Does peak oxygen pulse complement peak oxygen uptake in risk stratifying patients with heart failure? Am J Cardiol 2009;104(4):554–8.

26. Bailey CS, Wooster LT, Buswell M, et al. Post-exercise oxygen uptake recovery delay: a novel index of impaired cardiac reserve capacity in heart failure. JACC Heart failure 2018;6(4):329–39.

27. Cohen-Solal A, Laperche T, Morvan D, et al. Prolonged kinetics of recovery of oxygen consumption after maximal graded exercise in patients with chronic heart failure. Analysis with gas exchange measurements and NMR spectroscopy. Circulation 1995;91(12):2924–32.

28. Nanas S, Nanas J, Kassiotis C, et al. Early recovery of oxygen kinetics after submaximal exercise test predicts functional capacity in patients with chronic heart failure. Eur J Heart Fail 2001;3(6):685–92.

29. Lewis GD, Shah RV, Pappagianopolas PP, et al. Determinants of ventilatory efficiency in heart failure: the role of right ventricular performance and pulmonary vascular tone. Circ Heart Fail 2008;1(4): 227–33.

30. Corra U, Pistono M, Mezzani A, et al. Sleep and exertional periodic breathing in chronic heart failure: prognostic importance and interdependence. Circulation 2006;113(1):44–50.

31. Sun XG, Hansen JE, Beshai JF, et al. Oscillatory breathing and exercise gas exchange abnormalities prognosticate early mortality and morbidity in heart failure. J Am Coll Cardiol 2010;55(17): 1814–23.

32. Murphy RM, Shah RV, Malhotra R, et al. Exercise oscillatory ventilation in systolic heart failure: an indicator of impaired hemodynamic response to exercise. Circulation 2011;124(13):1442–51.

33. Forman DE, Guazzi M, Myers J, et al. Ventilatory power: a novel index that enhances prognostic assessment of patients with heart failure. Circ Heart Fail 2012;5(5):621–6.

34. Cohen-Solal A, Tabet JY, Logeart D, et al. A non-invasively determined surrogate of cardiac power ('circulatory power') at peak exercise is a powerful prognostic factor in chronic heart failure. Eur Heart J 2002;23(10):806–14.

35. Williams SG, Tzeng BH, Barker D, et al. Comparison and relation of indirect and direct dynamic indexes of cardiac pumping capacity in chronic heart failure. Am J Cardiol 2005;96(8):1149–50.

36. Namasivayam M, Lau ES, Zern EK, et al. Exercise blood pressure in heart failure with preserved and reduced ejection fraction. JACC Heart failure 2022; 10(4):278–86.

37. Myers J, Arena R, Dewey F, et al. A cardiopulmonary exercise testing score for predicting outcomes in patients with heart failure. Am Heart J 2008;156(6): 1177–83.

38. Jain CC, Borlaug BA. Performance and interpretation of invasive hemodynamic exercise testing. Chest 2020;158(5):2119–29.

39. Lewis GD, Houstis NE. The upsurge in exercise hemodynamic measurements in heart failure with preserved ejection fraction. JACC Heart failure 2019; 7(4):333–5.

40. Houstis NE, Eisman AS, Pappagianopoulos PP, et al. Exercise intolerance in heart failure with preserved ejection fraction: diagnosing and ranking its causes using personalized O(2) pathway analysis. Circulation 2018;137(2):148–61.

41. Campain J, Giverts I, Schoenicke MW, et al. Characterization and prognostic implications of respirophasic variation in invasive hemodynamic measurements at rest and with exercise. J Card Fail 2024;30(6):843–7.

42. Roul G, Moulichon ME, Bareiss P, et al. Prognostic factors of chronic heart failure in NYHA class II or III: value of invasive exercise haemodynamic data. Eur Heart J 1995;16(10):1387–98.

43. Lunney JR, Lynn J, Foley DJ, et al. Patterns of functional decline at the end of life. JAMA 2003;289(18): 2387–92.

44. Pritchard A, Burns P, Correia J, et al. ARTP statement on cardiopulmonary exercise testing 2021. BMJ Open Respir Res 2021;8(1). https://doi.org/10.1136/bmjresp-2021-001121.

45. Hansen JE, Sue DY, Wasserman K. Predicted values for clinical exercise testing. The American review of respiratory disease 1984;129(2 Pt 2):S49–55.

46. Gitt AK, Wasserman K, Kilkowski C, et al. Exercise anaerobic threshold and ventilatory efficiency identify heart failure patients for high risk of early death. Circulation 2002;106(24):3079–84.

47. Nayor M, Houstis NE, Namasivayam M, et al. Impaired exercise tolerance in heart failure with preserved ejection fraction: quantification of multiorgan system reserve capacity. JACC Heart failure 2020; 8(8):605–17.

48. Mancini DM, Eisen H, Kussmaul W, et al. Value of peak exercise oxygen consumption for optimal timing of cardiac transplantation in ambulatory patients with heart failure. Circulation 1991;83(3):778–86.

49. Peled Y, Ducharme A, Kittleson M, et al. International society for heart and Lung transplantation guidelines for the evaluation and care of cardiac transplant candidates-2024. J Heart Lung Transplant 2024. https://doi.org/10.1016/j.healun.2024.05.010.

50. Nadruz W Jr, West E, Sengeløv M, et al. Prognostic value of cardiopulmonary exercise testing in heart failure with reduced, midrange, and preserved ejection fraction. J Am Heart Assoc 2017;6(11). https://doi.org/10.1161/jaha.117.006000.

51. Guazzi M, Raimondo R, Vicenzi M, et al. Exercise oscillatory ventilation may predict sudden cardiac death in heart failure patients. J Am Coll Cardiol 2007;50(4):299–308.

52. Myers J, Gujja P, Neelagaru S, et al. End-tidal CO2 pressure and cardiac performance during exercise in heart failure. Med Sci Sports Exerc 2009;41(1): 19–25.

53. Osada N, Chaitman BR, Miller LW, et al. Cardiopulmonary exercise testing identifies low risk patients with heart failure and severely impaired exercise capacity considered for heart transplantation. J Am Coll Cardiol 1998;31(3):577–82.

54. Mancini D, LeJemtel T, Aaronson K. Peak VO(2): a simple yet enduring standard. Circulation 2000; 101(10):1080–2.

55. Vainshelboim B, Kokkinos P, Myers J. Prognostic value and clinical usefulness of the hemodynamic gain index in men. Am J Cardiol 2019;124(4):644–9.

56. Vainshelboim B, Kokkinos P, Myers J. Hemodynamic gain index in women: a validation study. Int J Cardiol 2020;308:15–9.

57. Agostoni P, Corrà U, Cattadori G, et al. Metabolic exercise test data combined with cardiac and kidney indexes, the MECKI score: a multiparametric approach to heart failure prognosis. Int J Cardiol 2013;167(6):2710–8.

58. Lala A, Shah KB, Lanfear DE, et al. Predictive value of cardiopulmonary exercise testing parameters in ambulatory advanced heart failure. JACC Heart failure 2021;9(3):226–36.

59. Chomsky DB, Lang CC, Rayos GH, et al. Hemodynamic exercise testing. A valuable tool in the selection of cardiac transplantation candidates. Circulation 1996;94(12):3176–83.

60. Lang CC, Karlin P, Haythe J, et al. Peak cardiac power output, measured noninvasively, is a powerful predictor of outcome in chronic heart failure. Circ Heart Fail 2009;2(1):33–8.

61. Eisman AS, Shah RV, Dhakal BP, et al. Pulmonary capillary wedge pressure patterns during exercise predict exercise capacity and incident heart failure. Circulation Heart failure 2018;11(5):e004750.

62. Ho JE, Zern EK, Wooster L, et al. Differential clinical profiles, exercise responses, and outcomes associated with existing HFpEF definitions. Circulation 2019;140(5):353–65.

63. Wilson JR, Hanamanthu S, Chomsky DB, et al. Relationship between exertional symptoms and functional capacity in patients with heart failure. J Am Coll Cardiol 1999;33(7):1943–7.

64. Birks EJ, Tansley PD, Hardy J, et al. Left ventricular assist device and drug therapy for the reversal of heart failure. N Engl J Med 2006;355(18):1873–84.

65. Steiner J, Wiafe S, Camuso J, et al. Predicting success: left ventricular assist device explantation evaluation protocol using comprehensive cardiopulmonary exercise testing. Circ Heart Fail 2017;10(1). https://doi.org/10.1161/circheartfailure.116.003694.

66. Beaver WL, Wasserman K, Whipp BJ. A new method for detecting anaerobic threshold by gas exchange. J Appl Physiol 1986;60(6):2020–7.

67. Kremser CB, O'Toole MF, Leff AR. Oscillatory hyperventilation in severe congestive heart failure secondary to idiopathic dilated cardiomyopathy or to ischemic cardiomyopathy. Am J Cardiol 1987;59(8):900–5.

68. Taivassalo T, Abbott A, Wyrick P, Haller RG. Venous oxygen levels during aerobic forearm exercise:an index of impaired oxidative metabolism in mitochondrial myopathy. Ann Neurol 2002;51(1):38–44.

69. Dhakal BP, Malhotra R, Murphy RM, et al. Mechanisms of exercise intolerance in heart failure with preserved ejection fraction: the role of abnormal peripheral oxygen extraction. Circ Heart Fail 2015;8(2):286–94.

70. Guazzi M, Arena R, Halle M, et al. 2016 Focused update: clinical recommendations for cardiopulmonary exercise testing data assessment in specific patient populations. Circulation. 2016;133(24):e694–711.

71. Borghi-Silva A, Labate V, Arena R, et al. Exercise ventilatory power in heart failure patients: functional phenotypes definition by combining cardiopulmonary exercise testing with stress echocardiography. Int J Cardiol 2014;176(3):1348–9.

72. Del Buono MG, Arena R, Borlaug BA, et al. Exercise intolerance in patients with heart failure: JACC state-of-the-art review. J Am Coll Cardiol 2019;73(17):2209–25.

Cardiopulmonary Exercise Testing in Pulmonary Hypertension

Kostiantyn Dmytriiev, MD[a], Michael K. Stickland, PhD[b,c],
Jason Weatherald, MD, MSc[a],*

KEYWORDS

- Pulmonary arterial hypertension • PAH • Cardiopulmonary exercise test • CPET • Invasive CPET

KEY POINTS

- The cardiopulmonary exercise test (CPET) can provide critical information about exercise tolerance, dyspnea, and pathophysiology of different pulmonary vascular diseases.
- CPET is crucial in assessing treatment response and prognosis in pulmonary arterial hypertension.
- Low peak oxygen consumption and ventilatory inefficiency combined with low partial end-tidal pressure of carbon dioxide are typical responses in pulmonary arterial hypertension.
- Some patients with PAH can demonstrate altered breathing mechanics, like dynamic hyperinflation, which can contribute to dyspnea and exercise tolerance.

INTRODUCTION

Pulmonary hypertension (PH) is a disease with diverse causes currently classified into 5 groups according to the common pathophysiological features, pulmonary vascular hemodynamics, and management.[1] Pulmonary arterial hypertension (PAH; group 1) is a chronic progressive pulmonary vascular disease characterized by vasoconstriction and proliferative vascular remodeling, including arteriolar muscularization and plexiform lesions, primarily affecting precapillary arterioles,[2–4] which lead to elevated pressure in the pulmonary arteries.[5] Patients with PAH have isolated precapillary PH, defined as mean pulmonary arterial pressure (mPAP) greater than 20 mm Hg, pulmonary artery wedge pressure (PAWP) 15 mm Hg or less, and pulmonary vascular resistance (PVR) greater than 2 Wood units.[1] An estimated prevalence of PAH ranges from 15 to 50 cases per million in Europe and the United States.[5,6] The 5 year survival rate in a Canadian PAH cohort was 56.0%,[7] comparable to survivability in all types of cancer.[8] The PAH population is heterogeneous, with female individuals demonstrating twice as high an incidence of hereditary PAH as compared to male individuals, while male individuals with PAH are typically diagnosed at an older age.[9] Hence, the purpose of this article is to review the mechanisms of exercise intolerance in PAH, and explain the role of cardiopulmonary exercise testing (CPET) in the clinical evaluation and prognosis of patients with PAH.

DISCUSSION

Mechanisms of Exercise Intolerance in Pulmonary Arterial Hypertension

Exertional dyspnea and exercise intolerance are cardinal features of PAH, with multiple factors

[a] Division of Pulmonary Medicine, Department of Medicine, University of Alberta, 3-110 Clinical Sciences Building, 11302 83 Avenue Northwest, Edmonton, Alberta T6G 2G3, Canada; [b] Division of Pulmonary Medicine, Department of Medicine, University of Alberta, 3-110 Clinical Sciences Building, 11302 83 Avenue Northwest, Edmonton, Alberta T6G 2G3, Canada; [c] G.F. MacDonald Centre for Lung Health, Covenant Health, 11111 Jasper Avenue, Edmonton, AB T5K 0L4, Canada
* Corresponding author.
E-mail address: weathera@ualberta.ca

Heart Failure Clin 21 (2025) 51–61
https://doi.org/10.1016/j.hfc.2024.05.002
1551-7136/25/© 2024 Elsevier Inc. All rights reserved, including those for text and data mining, AI training, and similar technologies.

potentially contributing to dyspnea.[10–13] The hallmark feature contributing to dyspnea and exercise intolerance in PAH is an exaggerated ventilatory response to exercise, as measured by high minute ventilation relative to carbon dioxide production ($\dot{V}_E/\dot{V}CO_2$).[10,14] The high $\dot{V}_E/\dot{V}CO_2$ originates from various sources that are secondary to pulmonary vascular remodeling: (1) ventilation-perfusion inequalities ($\dot{V}_A/\dot{Q}$ mismatch),[15] (2) low alveolar-capillary diffusion capacity, (3) impaired ability to increase right ventricular (RV) cardiac output with exercise, and (4) skeletal muscle dysfunction and deconditioning.[10,14] All these factors, combined with abnormal ventilatory mechanics, lead to higher perceived dyspnea and lower exercise tolerance (**Fig. 1**).[14]

Cardiac Adaptation and Abnormal Response to Exercise in Pulmonary Arterial Hypertension

Obliterative changes in the pulmonary arteries lead to increased PVR, high pulmonary artery shear stress,[16] and an increased afterload on the RV.[4,17] In response to this greater afterload, the RV undergoes hypertrophy, dilation, fat deposition, and fibrosis with disease progression.[18] As the RV has a lower muscle mass than the left ventricle, increases in afterload will significantly impact the ability of the RV to increase cardiac output during exercise.[10] Increased RV mass, RV microvascular dysfunction, and increased RV end-diastolic filling pressure are associated with RV ischemia.[19] These can also contribute to RV dyssynchrony, which can be a product of mechanical[20] and electrical delay.[21]

The alterations in baseline RV structure and increased afterload during exercise lead to an insufficient ability to augment stroke volume with exercise in patients with PH,[22] and therefore, increases in cardiac output with exercise are predominantly due to increases in heart rate.[23] The impaired ability of the RV to adapt to increased afterload results in RV–pulmonary arterial (RV–PA) uncoupling.[24,25] RV–PA coupling is a relationship between RV contractility and RV afterload and represent the

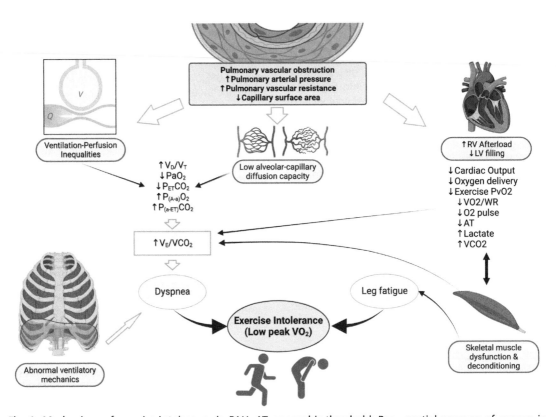

Fig. 1. Mechanisms of exercise intolerance in PAH. AT, anaerobic threshold; Pa_{O_2}, partial pressure of oxygen in arterial blood; $P_{(A\text{-}a)}O_2$, alveolar-arterial oxygen gradient; $P_{(a\text{-}ET)}CO_2$, arterial to end-tidal partial pressure of carbon dioxide; $P_{ET}CO_2$, partial pressure of carbon dioxide at the end of the exhalation; PvO_2, mixed venous oxygen tension; O_2, oxygen; $\dot{V}_E/\dot{V}CO_2$, high minute ventilation relative to carbon dioxide production; V_D/V_T, dead space to tidal volume ratio; VCO_2, carbon dioxide production; $\dot{V}O_2$, peak oxygen consumption; WR, work rate. (Figure created with BioRender.com.)

ability of RV function to properly match PVR.[26] It is calculated as a ratio of RV contractility measured by maximal ventricular elastance and arterial elastance as a product of PVR and heart rate. Thus, the RV–PA coupling can be reduced when RV contractility drops or afterload increases.[27] RV–PA coupling reflects disease severity[28] and has been shown to be superior to RV ejection fraction in predicting clinical worsening in PAH.[29] Thus, assessment of RV–PA coupling can help to identify high-risk patients as well as predict outcomes.

Sjogren and colleagues demonstrated lower left atrial and left ventricular (LV) volumes in PAH compared to controls,[30] which persist with exercise.[22] This reflects both ventricular interdependence and the inability of the RV to properly increase cardiac output with exercise, which can cause a reduction in LV filling pressures and systemic blood pressure fluctuations.[11,31] Thus, the assessment of cardiac response to exercise is an important part in the evaluation of patients with PAH, as this can aid evaluation and risk stratify patients with PAH.

Skeletal Muscle Dysfunction in Pulmonary Arterial Hypertension

Another critical factor that leads to exercise intolerance in patients with PAH is decreased oxygen extraction in the skeletal muscles,[32] which comes from 2 different sources: skeletal muscle dysfunction and/or deconditioning[33,34] and muscle capillary rarefaction.[35,36] The decreased skeletal muscle extraction,[37] combined with reduced O_2 delivery,[38] leads to peripheral muscle metaboreflex stimulation, further increasing exercise minute ventilation (and $\dot{V}_E/\dot{V}CO_2$) and perceived dyspnea in people with PAH.[12]

Abnormal Pulmonary Function and Dynamic Hyperinflation in Pulmonary Arterial Hypertension

Patients with PAH usually have normal pulmonary function tests and are likely to demonstrate normal breathing patterns during exercise (**Fig. 2**A), but some can exhibit restrictive[39] or obstructive[40] patterns, or a combination of both during pulmonary function tests.[1] These impairments in lung function can contribute to exercise intolerance in PAH and partially explain the development of dynamic hyperinflation (DH) that is present in some patients with PAH.[41,42] DH is a progressive reduction in inspiratory capacity (IC) due to an increase in end-expiratory lung volume (EELV) during exercise that leads to the decrease of end-inspiratory lung volume (EILV) and inspiratory reserve volume (IRV), a phenomenon classically seen in patients with

airflow obstruction, such as chronic obstructive pulmonary disease (**Fig. 2**B). The consequence of DH is that tidal breathing occurs closer to the total lung capacity (ie, at higher lung volumes), which requires greater work of breathing[43] and increases the perception of dyspnea.[42] Moreover, a progressive increase in EELV leads to decreased tidal volume (V_T), so ventilation is maintained or increased primarily through the breathing frequency.[43] Unlike PAH, a significant proportion of patients with LV failure with reduced or preserved ejection fraction have exercise oscillatory ventilation (EOV). EOV is a periodic breathing pattern characterized by cyclic variation in ventilation, similar to Cheyne–Stokes breathing, but without interposed apnea, which is not observed in patients with PAH (**Fig. 2**C).[44] Thus, the presence of EOV during CPET can be helpful in the differential diagnosis and distinguishing between PAH and LV dysfunction.

Abnormal Ventilatory Response to Exercise in Pulmonary Arterial Hypertension

The pathologic changes in the pulmonary circulation also lead to the inefficient ventilatory response to exercise as represented by high $\dot{V}_E/\dot{V}CO_2$, a hallmark feature of pulmonary vascular diseases. High $\dot{V}_E/\dot{V}CO_2$ is conditioned by low P_{aCO_2} and/or high dead space[45] ventilation (ie, V_D/V_T; Equation 1). Remodeling of the arterial bed in PAH[46] leads to ventilation/perfusion inequality,[14] and as a consequence, high V_D/V_T,[45] which is evident even in mild PAH.[47] A second important reason for high $\dot{V}_E/\dot{V}CO_2$ is low P_{aCO_2} at rest and during exercise,[48,49] likely due to enhanced chemosensitivity and low P_{aCO_2} setpoint,[50] resulting in increased neural drive to breathe,[51] and higher minute ventilation for a given $\dot{V}CO_2$ output.[14] Chemosensitivity and calculations of V_D/V_T in cardiopulmonary diseases are discussed in detail elsewhere.[52–54]

$$\frac{\dot{V}_E}{\dot{V}_{CO_2}} = \frac{k}{P_{aCO_2} \times \left(1 - \frac{V_D}{V_T}\right)} \quad \text{Equation 1}$$

Why Measuring Exercise Capacity Is Important in Pulmonary Arterial Hypertension

Progressive dyspnea with exertion significantly affects quality of life (QoL) by reducing physical function.[55] In fact, everyday activities like doing laundry, cooking, or walking can be above the anaerobic threshold in many patients with PAH.[12] Patients with PAH demonstrate a reduction in all domains of QoL questionnaires with a greater reduction in domains related to physical functioning,[55–58] with

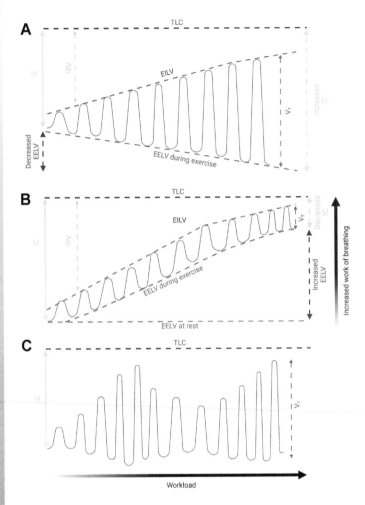

Fig. 2. Change in tidal breathing with increasing workload: (*A*) Pattern of normal breathing during exercise is characterized by the gradual decrease of EELV and increase of IC due to the increased V_T; (*B*) Pattern of breathing during exercise in DH is characterized by the gradual increase of EELV and decrease of IC, that result in lower V_T and higher breathing frequency, and as a consequence in higher work of breathing; (*C*) EOV—pattern seen during exercise in heart failure. EELV, end-expiratory lung volume; EILV, end-inspiratory lung volume; IC, inspiratory capacity; IRV, inspiratory reserve volume; TLC, total lung capacity; V_T, tidal volume. (Figure created with BioRender.com.)

the physical component score showing an ability to predict mortality in PAH,[58,59] and disease progression.[60] Both peak oxygen consumption ($\dot{V}O_{2peak}$) measured by CPET and exercise capacity measured by the 6 minute walking distance (6MWD) are independent predictors of the QoL.[61] In a series of studies, Matura and colleagues identified that shortness of breath during exercise and fatigue were the most often contributing symptoms to the reduced QoL in patients with PAH,[62] and lower QoL is found in patients with worse cardiopulmonary symptoms.[63]

As exercise intolerance is the main symptom in patients with PAH, its assessment is crucial to inform risk stratification and management. The importance of exercise testing in this population has been highlighted in all PH guidelines and expert statements over the last 15 years.[1,64–66] Earlier guidelines stratified patients into risk groups according to only 6MWD or oxygen consumption ($\dot{V}O_2$),[64–66] while risk assessment scales were developed and included in the most recent guidelines published.[1] The current PAH risk

assessment scale includes 6MWD, $\dot{V}O_{2peak}$ and the slope of $\dot{V}_E/\dot{V}CO_2$ obtained from CPET, and right heart catheterization (RHC) data that reflect cardiopulmonary function, such as right atrial pressure, cardiac index, stroke volume index, and mixed venous oxygen saturation (SvO_2).[1] Thus, CPET can provide valuable information on the exercise capacity and causes of exercise intolerance, which is necessary for the clinical management of patients with PAH.

It is also important to mention that several alternative methods to measure exercise capacity have been proposed. For example, a 1 minute sit-to-stand test showed a good correlation with 6MWD in patients with PAH and was recently proposed as an alternative to 6MWT.[67] Robertson and colleagues compared a 1 minute walking test performed remotely with the 6MWT performed in the clinics and found a strong association between the 2 along with similar predictive capabilities.[68] Studies demonstrated that these tests are safe, and patients with PAH and chronic thromboembolic PH[69] and interstitial lung diseases[68] are willing to perform this test at home, opening possibilities for the remote monitoring of exercise capacity in these patients. Another alternative that showed good associations with both 6MWT and $\dot{V}O_{2peak}$ was the incremental shuttle walking test,[70] which was also correlated with mortality in PAH.[70,71] While these tests demonstrate good predictive value and are cheap and easy to perform, they provide only limited information about underlying pathophysiology or mechanisms of exercise intolerance.[72]

Cardiopulmonary Exercise Test Abnormalities in Patients with Pulmonary Arterial Hypertension

Abnormalities in CPET parameters in PAH come from multiple cardiopulmonary and peripheral derangements described in detail in earlier sections. Patients with PAH demonstrate reduced exercise tolerance as measured by reduced peak work rate (WR), oxygen consumption, $\dot{V}O_2$/WR slope, and $\dot{V}O_2$ efficiency slope.[73] Impaired circulatory response to exercise is evident by decreases in peak heart rate, oxygen pulse, and peak circulatory power.[74] Abnormalities in gas exchange include arterial desaturation, high $\dot{V}_E/\dot{V}CO_2$ slope, and high nadir $\dot{V}_E/\dot{V}CO_2$ and low end-tidal CO_2 pressure ($P_{ET}CO_2$).[75]

Cardiopulmonary Exercise Test Parameters Linked to Prognosis in Pulmonary Arterial Hypertension

The 6MWT is used more often than CPET to predict mortality risk and treatment efficacy in clinical settings and clinical trials. There is a larger body of knowledge regarding 6MWD in PAH compared to CPET,[76] nevertheless, several studies demonstrated additional benefits of CPET at predicting mortality in PAH.[77,78] Patients with PAH, as well as with many other cardiopulmonary diseases, demonstrate reduced $\dot{V}O_2$ at peak exercise[79] and low anaerobic threshold,[80] which are associated with poorer clinical outcomes.[81] As discussed earlier, patients with PAH often exhibit an exaggerated ventilatory response to exercise with high $\dot{V}_E/\dot{V}CO_2$. In general, higher $\dot{V}_E/\dot{V}CO_2$ slope and higher $\dot{V}_E/\dot{V}CO_2$ nadir are associated with more severe disease and worse outcomes.[14,73] A $\dot{V}_E/\dot{V}CO_2$ slope greater than 44 indicates a high-risk assessment parameter in the current PH guidelines, whereas a $\dot{V}_E/\dot{V}CO_2$ slope less than 36 is associated with a low-risk status[1] **(Table 1)**.

$\dot{V}O_2$ efficiency slope is an additional parameter covered in some research articles that can provide additional predictive value in PAH.[82,83] It is defined as the regression slope in equation $\dot{V}O_2 = a \times log10(V_E) + b$.[83] Similar to $\dot{V}_E/\dot{V}CO_2$, a high $\dot{V}O_2$ efficiency slope likely reflects altered ventilation/perfusion matching and can be derived from the CPET data from the relationship between $\dot{V}O_2$ and the logarithmic transformation of minute ventilation.[82,83] Patients with PAH demonstrate abnormal $\dot{V}O_2$ efficiency slope,[82,83] which was linked to the higher PAH-related mortality or need for atrial septostomy even after the adjustment for $\dot{V}O_2$, $\dot{V}_E/\dot{V}CO_2$, and $\dot{V}O_2$/WR slope.[84]

Cardiopulmonary Exercise Test in the Differential Diagnosis

$\dot{V}_E/\dot{V}CO_2$ can be used to screen for PAH or help to differentiate between different conditions. A

Table 1
Cardiopulmonary exercise test parameters that change in pulmonary arterial hypertension and their prognostic roles

Parameter	Important Cutoffs	Predictive Value
$\dot{V}O_2$ peak	>15 mL/min/kg or >65% pred 11–15 mL/min/kg or 35%–65% pred <11 mL/min/kg or <35% pred	*1 y mortality risk:* Low Intermediate High[1]
$\dot{V}_E/\dot{V}CO_2$ slope	<36 36–44 >44	*1 y mortality risk:* Low risk Intermediate risk High risk[1]
$\dot{V}O_2$ efficiency slope	$\leq$0.56 L/min	Higher mortality[82,83]
$\dot{V}_E/\dot{V}CO_2$ at anaerobic threshold (AT)	>54–55 at AT	Low survival[78,85–88]
$P_{ET}CO_2$ at AT	<35	High PAH probability[75]

$V_E/\dot{V}CO_2$ nadir greater than 35.5,[89] slope 39 or greater,[90] or a combination of $\dot{V}_E/\dot{V}CO_2$ slope greater than 33.9 with low $\dot{V}O_2$ ($\leq$14.1 mL/kg/min) and $P_{ET}CO_2$ ($\leq$27.2 mm Hg) had a high ability to discriminate patients with systemic sclerosis who had PAH.[91] Dumitrescu and colleagues demonstrated that $\dot{V}_E/\dot{V}CO_2$ nadir greater than 35.5 had 79.2% sensitivity and 82.9% specificity to detect PAH in patients with scleroderma, while a $\dot{V}_E/\dot{V}CO_2$ nadir greater than 45.5 had a positive predictive value of 100%.[89]

Discriminating PAH and chronic thromboembolic pulmonary hypertension (CTEPH) on CPET can be challenging as both conditions demonstrate an increase in $\dot{V}_E/\dot{V}CO_2$ and a reduction in $P_{ET}CO_2$.[14] Patients with CTEPH exhibit higher V_D/V_T ventilation that drives higher $\dot{V}_E/\dot{V}CO_2$ slope and $\dot{V}_E/\dot{V}CO_2$ at AT.[92,93] Akizuki and colleagues proposed distinguishing between 2 conditions by a postural change in $\dot{V}_E/\dot{V}CO_2$. Authors demonstrated that $\dot{V}_E/\dot{V}CO_2$ decreased in the supine position in PAH and increased in CTEPH, and $\Delta\dot{V}_E/\dot{V}CO_2$ greater than 0.8 had 78% sensitivity and 88% specificity in differentiating CTEPH from PAH.[94]

Distinguishing between PAH and left heart failure, especially heart failure with preserved ejection fraction (HFpEF), can be clinically challenging as both conditions have normal LV systolic function on echocardiography, have similar symptoms, and demonstrate limitations during exercise. Patients with PAH generally demonstrate higher $\dot{V}_E/\dot{V}CO_2$ slopes and lower peak $\dot{V}O_2$ than patients with HFpEF and heart failure with reduced ejection fraction.[80] The main feature that discriminates between these conditions is EOV, which is present only in patients with left heart failure and not observed in PAH (see **Fig. 2**C).[95]

RHC during CPET (invasive CPET, or iCPET) can be a valuable method to provide clarity in cases with normal resting hemodynamics, comorbidities, or controversial noninvasive data.[96] The normal response to exercise includes a reduction of PVR due to the pulmonary vasodilation and capillary recruitment, combined with the greater increase in CO and PAWP, this results in the increase of mPAP. The mPAP increases proportionally to increasing CO during exercise. The ratio of mPAP to CO, therefore, needs to be considered. The normal mPAP/CO increase during exercise is reported to be 0.5 to 3.0 mm Hg/L/min.[97] Impaired ability to recruit and/or distend the pulmonary vasculature leads to the steeper rise of mPAP/CO slope due to the insufficient reduction of PVR and/or higher increase in PAWP with exercise in pulmonary vascular diseases.[97] An abnormal mPAP/CO slope (>3 mm Hg/L/min) combined with normal resting mPAP was defined as exercise PH in the most recent guidelines.[1] An abnormal mPAP/CO slope is associated with lower $\dot{V}O_2$ and higher risk of cardiovascular hospitalizations and all-cause mortality in the population of patients with chronic exertional dyspnea,[98] and can help identify patients at higher risk of developing PAH as was demonstrated in connective tissue diseases[99] and asymptomatic bone morphogenetic protein receptor type 2 carriers.[100] In addition to that, abnormal mPAP/CO slope identified patients with PAH and CTEPH on optimized medical therapy at higher risk of mortality.[101] Performing iCPET during an RHC can help distinguish between the LV dysfunction and PAH. Patients with left heart disease usually have elevated PAWP of greater than 15 mm Hg at rest. However, in some cases, patients with left heart disease may have normal resting PAWP due to treatment with diuretics, though they typically exhibit an abnormal PAWP during exercise and a PAWP/CO slope greater than 2 mm Hg/L/min during exercise.[102] An increase in PAWP to greater than 25 mm Hg or PAWP/CO slope greater than 2 during exercise can be useful for identifying occult LV diastolic dysfunction and differentiating HFpEF from PAH when the diagnosis is unclear (**Table 2**).[102–104]

Cardiopulmonary Exercise Test in the Assessment of Treatment Response

CPET is widely used to assess the impact of therapeutic interventions across different pulmonary and cardiovascular conditions, including PAH.[106] It was demonstrated by Groepenhoff and colleagues that survivors with PAH had a higher change in peak $\dot{V}O_2$ following treatment initiation,[107] which can help to discriminate patients at higher risk of adverse outcomes. Hirashiki and colleagues also demonstrated that CPET-guided treatment goals with $\dot{V}O_2$ 15.0 mL/min/kg or greater and systolic blood pressure greater than 120 mm Hg helped to improve 3 year mortality

Table 2		
Important cutoffs of invasive cardiopulmonary exercise test parameters		
Parameter	**Important Cutoffs**	**Diagnostic Value**
mPAP/CO slope	>3 mm Hg/L/min	Exercise PH[1]
PAWP/CO slope	>2 mm Hg/L/min	LV diastolic dysfunction/HFpEF[1]
PAWP	>25 mm Hg	Cutoff for HFpEF diagnosis[105]

by 10%.[108] Thus, CPET can provide additional information after the treatment initiation and help further stratify patients according to their response to treatment.

SUMMARY

Patients with PAH demonstrate a broad spectrum of cardiopulmonary physiologic abnormalities that lead to reduced exercise capacity. CPET is the gold standard in assessing exercise tolerance. It can provide a valuable information to help discriminate between different pulmonary vascular diseases as well as for the diagnosis, prognosis, and treatment response assessment in PAH.

CLINICS CARE POINTS

- The CPET is useful in discriminating between conditions with reduced exercise tolerance.
- Inefficient ventilation (high $\dot{V}_E/\dot{V}CO_2$) combined with low $P_{ET}CO_2$ and low exercise capacity is typical for PAH and CTEPH.
- EOV can suggest a diagnosis of left heart dysfunction rather than PAH when the diagnosis is unclear.
- High $\dot{V}_E/\dot{V}CO_2$ can help to identify patients with pulmonary vascular contribution to exercise intolerance is a prognostic marker in patients with PAH and CTEPH.
- mPAP/CO slope with invasive CPET can help to identify patients at higher risk of developing PH and/or higher risk of hospitalization and mortality.

DISCLOSURE

K. Dmytriiev has nothing to disclose; M.K. Stickland has nothing to disclose, J. Weatherald has received grants or contracts to his institution from Astra Zeneca, Bayer, Janssen, Sanofi, and Merck; consulting fees from Janssen and Merck; honoraria from Janssen and Merck; advisory board payments from Janssen and Merck, payment for expert testimony from Sprigings Intellectual Property Law; travel support from Janssen; participation on Data Safety and Monitoring Board for the Université de Laval; and has unpaid leadership role at the Pulmonary Hypertension Association of Canada.

REFERENCES

1. Humbert M, Kovacs G, Hoeper MM, et al. 2022 ESC/ERS Guidelines for the diagnosis and treatment of pulmonary hypertension: Developed by the task force for the diagnosis and treatment of pulmonary hypertension of the European Society of Cardiology (ESC) and the European Respiratory Society (ERS). Endorsed by the International Society for Heart and Lung Transplantation (ISHLT) and the European Reference Network on rare respiratory diseases (ERN-LUNG). Eur Heart J 2022; 43(38):3618–731.
2. Liang S, Desai AA, Black SM, et al. Cytokines, Chemokines, and Inflammation in Pulmonary Arterial Hypertension. Adv Exp Med Biol 2021;1303:275–303.
3. Shah AJ, Vorla M, Kalra DK. Molecular pathways in pulmonary arterial hypertension. Int J Mol Sci 2022; 23(17):10001.
4. Hassoun PM. Pulmonary arterial hypertension. N Engl J Med 2021;385(25):2361–76.
5. Ruopp NF, Cockrill BA. Diagnosis and treatment of pulmonary arterial hypertension: a review. JAMA 2022;327(14):1379–91.
6. Beshay S, Sahay S, Humbert M. Evaluation and management of pulmonary arterial hypertension. Respir Med 2020;171:106099.
7. Zelt JGE, Sugarman J, Weatherald J, et al. Mortality trends in pulmonary arterial hypertension in Canada: a temporal analysis of survival per ESC/ ERS guideline era. Eur Respir J 2022;59(6).
8. Ellison LF. The cancer survival index: Measuring progress in cancer survival to help evaluate cancer control efforts in Canada. Health Rep 2021;32(9): 14–26.
9. Lau EMT, Giannoulatou E, Celermajer DS, et al. Epidemiology and treatment of pulmonary arterial hypertension. Nat Rev Cardiol 2017;14(10):603–14.
10. Neder JA, Phillips DB, O'Donnell DE, et al. Excess ventilation and exertional dyspnoea in heart failure and pulmonary hypertension. Eur Respir J 2022; 60(5):2200144.
11. Laveneziana P, Weatherald J. Pulmonary vascular disease and cardiopulmonary exercise testing. Front Physiol 2020;11:964.
12. Malenfant S, Lebret M, Breton-Gagnon É, et al. Exercise intolerance in pulmonary arterial hypertension: insight into central and peripheral pathophysiological mechanisms. Eur Respir Rev 2021; 30(160):200284.
13. Tran DL, Lau EMT, Celermajer DS, et al. Pathophysiology of exercise intolerance in pulmonary arterial hypertension. Respirology 2018;23(2):148–59.
14. Weatherald J, Philipenko B, Montani D, et al. Ventilatory efficiency in pulmonary vascular diseases. Eur Respir Rev 2021;30(161):200214.
15. Suga K, Tokuda O, Okada M, et al. Assessment of cross-sectional lung ventilation-perfusion imbalance in primary and passive pulmonary hypertension with automated V/Q SPECT. Nucl Med Commun 2010;31(7):673–81.

16. Fukui S, Ogo T, Goto Y, et al. Exercise intolerance and ventilatory inefficiency improve early after balloon pulmonary angioplasty in patients with inoperable chronic thromboembolic pulmonary hypertension. Int J Cardiol 2015;180:66–8.

17. Naeije R, Manes A. The right ventricle in pulmonary arterial hypertension. Eur Respir Rev 2014;23(134):476–87.

18. Vonk Noordegraaf A, Chin KM, Haddad F, et al. Pathophysiology of the right ventricle and of the pulmonary circulation in pulmonary hypertension: an update. Eur Respir J 2019;53(1):1801900.

19. Gómez A, Bialostozky D, Zajarias A, et al. Right ventricular ischemia in patients with primary pulmonary hypertension. J Am Coll Cardiol 2001;38(4):1137–42.

20. Marcus JT, Gan CT, Zwanenburg JJ, et al. Interventricular mechanical asynchrony in pulmonary arterial hypertension: left-to-right delay in peak shortening is related to right ventricular overload and left ventricular underfilling. J Am Coll Cardiol 2008;51(7):750–7.

21. Hill AC, Maxey DM, Rosenthal DN, et al. Electrical and mechanical dyssynchrony in pediatric pulmonary hypertension. J Heart Lung Transplant 2012;31(8):825–30.

22. Nootens M, Wolfkiel CJ, Chomka EV, et al. Understanding right and left ventricular systolic function and interactions at rest and with exercise in primary pulmonary hypertension. Am J Cardiol 1995;75(5):374–7.

23. Provencher S, Chemla D, Hervé P, et al. Heart rate responses during the 6-minute walk test in pulmonary arterial hypertension. Eur Respir J 2006;27(1):114–20.

24. Oakland H, Joseph P, Naeije R, et al. Arterial load and right ventricular-vascular coupling in pulmonary hypertension. J Appl Physiol (1985) 2021;131(1):424–33.

25. Bellofiore A, Dinges E, Naeije R, et al. Reduced haemodynamic coupling and exercise are associated with vascular stiffening in pulmonary arterial hypertension. Heart (British Cardiac Society) 2017;103(6):421–7.

26. He Q, Lin Y, Zhu Y, et al. Clinical Usefulness of Right Ventricle-Pulmonary Artery Coupling in Cardiovascular Disease. J Clin Med 2023;12(7):2526.

27. Naeije R, Chesler N. Pulmonary circulation at exercise. Compr Physiol 2012;2(1):711–41.

28. Li Y, Guo D, Gong J, et al. Right Ventricular Function and Its Coupling With Pulmonary Circulation in Precapillary Pulmonary Hypertension: A Three-Dimensional Echocardiographic Study. Front Cardiovasc Med 2021;8:690606.

29. Hsu S, Simpson CE, Houston BA, et al. Multi-Beat Right Ventricular-Arterial Coupling Predicts Clinical Worsening in Pulmonary Arterial Hypertension. J Am Heart Assoc 2020;9(10):e016031.

30. Sjögren H, Kjellström B, Bredfelt A, et al. Underfilling decreases left ventricular function in pulmonary arterial hypertension. Int J Cardiovasc Imaging 2021;37(5):1745–55.

31. Hardegree EL, Sachdev A, Fenstad ER, et al. Impaired left ventricular mechanics in pulmonary arterial hypertension: identification of a cohort at high risk. Circulation Heart failure 2013;6(4):748–55.

32. Barbosa PB, Ferreira EM, Arakaki JS, et al. Kinetics of skeletal muscle O2 delivery and utilization at the onset of heavy-intensity exercise in pulmonary arterial hypertension. Eur J Appl Physiol 2011;111(8):1851–61.

33. Batt J, Ahmed SS, Correa J, et al. Skeletal muscle dysfunction in idiopathic pulmonary arterial hypertension. Am J Respir Cell Mol Biol 2014;50(1):74–86.

34. Marra AM, Arcopinto M, Bossone E, et al. Pulmonary arterial hypertension-related myopathy: an overview of current data and future perspectives. Nutr Metabol Cardiovasc Dis 2015;25(2):131–9.

35. Malenfant S, Potus F, Mainguy V, et al. Impaired Skeletal Muscle Oxygenation and Exercise Tolerance in Pulmonary Hypertension. Med Sci Sports Exerc 2015;47(11):2273–82.

36. Potus F, Malenfant S, Graydon C, et al. Impaired angiogenesis and peripheral muscle microcirculation loss contribute to exercise intolerance in pulmonary arterial hypertension. Am J Respir Crit Care Med 2014;190(3):318–28.

37. Meyer FJ, Lossnitzer D, Kristen AV, et al. Respiratory muscle dysfunction in idiopathic pulmonary arterial hypertension. Eur Respir J 2005;25(1):125–30.

38. Waxman AB. Exercise physiology and pulmonary arterial hypertension. Prog Cardiovasc Dis 2012;55(2):172–9.

39. Sun XG, Hansen JE, Oudiz RJ, et al. Pulmonary function in primary pulmonary hypertension. J Am Coll Cardiol 2003;41(6):1028–35.

40. Meyer FJ, Ewert R, Hoeper MM, et al. Peripheral airway obstruction in primary pulmonary hypertension. Thorax 2002;57(6):473–6.

41. Laveneziana P, Garcia G, Joureau B, et al. Dynamic respiratory mechanics and exertional dyspnoea in pulmonary arterial hypertension. Eur Respir J 2013;41(3):578–87.

42. Laveneziana P, Humbert M, Godinas L, et al. Inspiratory muscle function, dynamic hyperinflation and exertional dyspnoea in pulmonary arterial hypertension. Eur Respir J 2015;45(5):1495–8.

43. Stickland MK, Neder JA, Guenette JA, et al. Using cardiopulmonary exercise testing to understand dyspnea and exercise intolerance in respiratory disease. Chest 2022;161(6):1505–16.

44. Dhakal BP, Lewis GD. Exercise oscillatory ventilation: mechanisms and prognostic significance. World J Cardiol 2016;8(3):258–66.

45. Kizhakke Puliyakote AS, Prisk GK, Elliott AR, et al. The spatial-temporal dynamics of pulmonary blood flow are altered in pulmonary arterial hypertension. J Appl Physiol (1985) 2023;134(4): 969–79.

46. Dantzker DR, Bower JS. Mechanisms of gas exchange abnormality in patients with chronic obliterative pulmonary vascular disease. J Clin Invest 1979;64(4):1050–5.

47. Plantier L, Delclaux C. Increased physiological dead space at exercise is a marker of mild pulmonary or cardiovascular disease in dyspneic subjects. European clinical respiratory journal 2018; 5(1):1492842.

48. Hoeper MM, Pletz MW, Golpon H, et al. Prognostic value of blood gas analyses in patients with idiopathic pulmonary arterial hypertension. Eur Respir J 2007;29(5):944–50.

49. Weatherald J, Boucly A, Montani D, et al. Gas exchange and ventilatory efficiency during exercise in pulmonary vascular diseases. Arch Bronconeumol 2020;56(9):578–85.

50. Naeije R, van de Borne P. Clinical relevance of autonomic nervous system disturbances in pulmonary arterial hypertension. Eur Respir J 2009;34(4): 792–4.

51. Mitrouska I, Bolaki M, Vaporidi K, et al. Respiratory system as the main determinant of dyspnea in patients with pulmonary hypertension. Pulm Circ 2022;12(1):e12060.

52. Weatherald J, Sattler C, Garcia G, et al. Ventilatory response to exercise in cardiopulmonary disease: the role of chemosensitivity and dead space. Eur Respir J 2018;51(2):1700860.

53. Phillips DB, Collins SÉ, Stickland MK. Measurement and Interpretation of Exercise Ventilatory Efficiency. Front Physiol 2020;11.

54. Caiozzo VJ, Davis JA, Ellis JF, et al. A comparison of gas exchange indices used to detect the anaerobic threshold. J Appl Physiol Respir Environ Exerc Physiol 1982;53(5):1184–9.

55. Sarzyńska K, Świątoniowska-Lonc N, Dudek K, et al. Quality of life of patients with pulmonary arterial hypertension: a meta-analysis. Eur Rev Med Pharmacol Sci 2021;25(15):4983–98.

56. Gu S, Hu H, Dong H. Systematic review of health-related quality of life in patients with pulmonary arterial hypertension. Pharmacoeconomics 2016; 34(8):751–70.

57. Chen H, De Marco T, Kobashigawa EA, et al. Comparison of cardiac and pulmonary-specific quality-of-life measures in pulmonary arterial hypertension. Eur Respir J 2011;38(3):608–16.

58. Fernandes CJ, Martins BC, Jardim CV, et al. Quality of life as a prognostic marker in pulmonary arterial hypertension. Health Qual Life Outcome 2014;12: 130.

59. Chen YJ, Tu HP, Lee CL, et al. Comprehensive exercise capacity and quality of life assessments predict mortality in patients with pulmonary arterial hypertension. Acta Cardiol Sin 2019;35(1):55–64.

60. Arvanitaki A, Mouratoglou SA, Evangeliou A, et al. Quality of Life is Related to Haemodynamics in Precapillary Pulmonary Hypertension. Heart Lung Circ 2020;29(1):142–8.

61. Halank M, Einsle F, Lehman S, et al. Exercise capacity affects quality of life in patients with pulmonary hypertension. Lung 2013;191(4):337–43.

62. Matura LA, McDonough A, Carroll DL. Cluster analysis of symptoms in pulmonary arterial hypertension: a pilot study. Eur J Cardiovasc Nurs 2012; 11(1):51–61.

63. Matura LA, McDonough A, Hanlon AL, et al. Sleep disturbance, symptoms, psychological distress, and health-related quality of life in pulmonary arterial hypertension. Eur J Cardiovasc Nurs 2015; 14(5):423–30.

64. Galiè N, Hoeper MM, Humbert M, et al. Guidelines for the diagnosis and treatment of pulmonary hypertension. Eur Respir J 2009;34(6): 1219–63.

65. Galiè N, Humbert M, Vachiery JL, et al. 2015 ESC/ERS Guidelines for the diagnosis and treatment of pulmonary hypertension: The Joint Task Force for the Diagnosis and Treatment of Pulmonary Hypertension of the European Society of Cardiology (ESC) and the European Respiratory Society (ERS): Endorsed by: Association for European Paediatric and Congenital Cardiology (AEPC), International Society for Heart and Lung Transplantation (ISHLT). Eur Heart J 2016;37(1):67–119.

66. McLaughlin VV, Archer SL, Badesch DB, et al. ACCF/AHA 2009 Expert Consensus Document on Pulmonary Hypertension. Circulation 2009;119(16): 2250–94.

67. Pereira MC, Lima LNG, Moreira MM, et al. One minute sit-to-stand test as an alternative to measure functional capacity in patients with pulmonary arterial hypertension. J Bras Pneumol 2022;48(3): e20210483.

68. Robertson L, Newman J, Clayton S, et al. The digital 1-minute walk test: a new patient-centered cardiorespiratory endpoint. Am J Respir Crit Care Med 2024;209(6):753–6.

69. Keen C, Smith I, Hashmi-Greenwood M, et al. Pulmonary hypertension and measurement of exercise capacity remotely: evaluation of the 1-min sit-to-stand test (PERSPIRE) - a cohort study. ERJ open research 2023;9(1):00295–2022.

70. Billings CG, Lewis R, Hurdman JA, et al. The incremental shuttle walk test predicts mortality in non-group 1 pulmonary hypertension: results from the ASPIRE Registry. Pulm Circ 2019;9(2). 2045894019848649.

71. Lewis RA, Billings CG, Hurdman JA, et al. Maximal exercise testing using the incremental shuttle walking test can be used to risk-stratify patients with pulmonary arterial hypertension. Annals of the American Thoracic Society 2021;18(1):34–43.

72. Heresi GA, Dweik RA. Strengths and limitations of the six-minute-walk test: a model biomarker study in idiopathic pulmonary fibrosis. Am J Respir Crit Care Med 2011;183(9):1122–4.

73. Sun XG, Hansen JE, Oudiz RJ, et al. Exercise pathophysiology in patients with primary pulmonary hypertension. Circulation 2001;104(4):429–35.

74. Li X, Duan A, Jin Q, et al. Exercise feature and predictor of prognosis in patients with pulmonary artery stenosis-associated pulmonary hypertension. ESC heart failure 2022;9(6):4198–208.

75. Luo Q, Yu X, Zhao Z, et al. The value of cardiopulmonary exercise testing in the diagnosis of pulmonary hypertension. J Thorac Dis 2021;13(1): 178–88.

76. Farina S, Correale M, Bruno N, et al. The role of cardiopulmonary exercise tests in pulmonary arterial hypertension. Eur Respir Rev 2018;27(148): 170134.

77. Groepenhoff H, Vonk-Noordegraaf A, Boonstra A, et al. Exercise testing to estimate survival in pulmonary hypertension. Med Sci Sports Exerc 2008; 40(10):1725–32.

78. Schwaiblmair M, Faul C, von Scheidt W, et al. Ventilatory efficiency testing as prognostic value in patients with pulmonary hypertension. BMC Pulm Med 2012;12:23.

79. Sherman AE, Saggar R. Cardiopulmonary exercise testing in pulmonary arterial hypertension. Heart Failure Clin 2023;19(1):35–43.

80. Deboeck G, Niset G, Lamotte M, et al. Exercise testing in pulmonary arterial hypertension and in chronic heart failure. Eur Respir J 2004;23(5): 747–51.

81. Ross R, Blair SN, Arena R, et al. Importance of assessing cardiorespiratory fitness in clinical practice: a case for fitness as a clinical vital sign: a scientific statement from the american heart association. Circulation 2016;134(24):e653–99.

82. Baba R, Nagashima M, Goto M, et al. Oxygen uptake efficiency slope: A new index of cardiorespiratory functional reserve derived from the relation between oxygen uptake and minute ventilation during incremental exercise. J Am Coll Cardiol 1996; 28(6):1567–72.

83. Tan X, Yang W, Guo J, et al. Usefulness of decrease in oxygen uptake efficiency to identify gas exchange abnormality in patients with idiopathic pulmonary arterial hypertension. PLoS One 2014;9(6):e98889.

84. Ramos RP, Ota-Arakaki JS, Alencar MC, et al. Exercise oxygen uptake efficiency slope independently predicts poor outcome in pulmonary arterial hypertension. Eur Respir J 2014;43(5):1510–2.

85. Wensel R, Opitz CF, Anker SD, et al. Assessment of survival in patients with primary pulmonary hypertension: importance of cardiopulmonary exercise testing. Circulation 2002;106(3):319–24.

86. Deboeck G, Scoditti C, Huez S, et al. Exercise testing to predict outcome in idiopathic versus associated pulmonary arterial hypertension. Eur Respir J 2012;40(6):1410–9.

87. Ferreira EV, Ota-Arakaki JS, Ramos RP, et al. Optimizing the evaluation of excess exercise ventilation for prognosis assessment in pulmonary arterial hypertension. European Journal of Preventive Cardiology 2014;21(11):1409–19.

88. Khatri V, Neal JE, Burger CD, et al. Prognostication in pulmonary arterial hypertension with submaximal exercise testing. Diseases 2015;3(1):15–23.

89. Dumitrescu D, Nagel C, Kovacs G, et al. Cardiopulmonary exercise testing for detecting pulmonary arterial hypertension in systemic sclerosis. Heart (British Cardiac Society) 2017;103(10): 774–82.

90. Santaniello A, Casella R, Vicenzi M, et al. Cardiopulmonary exercise testing in a combined screening approach to individuate pulmonary arterial hypertension in systemic sclerosis. Rheumatology (Oxford, England) 2020;59(7):1581–6.

91. Bellan M, Giubertoni A, Piccinino C, et al. Cardiopulmonary Exercise Testing Is an Accurate Tool for the Diagnosis of Pulmonary Arterial Hypertension in Scleroderma Related Diseases. Pharmaceuticals 2021;14(4):342.

92. Zhai Z, Murphy K, Tighe H, et al. Differences in ventilatory inefficiency between pulmonary arterial hypertension and chronic thromboembolic pulmonary hypertension. Chest 2011;140(5):1284–91.

93. Scheidl SJ, Englisch C, Kovacs G, et al. Diagnosis of CTEPH versus IPAH using capillary to end-tidal carbon dioxide gradients. Eur Respir J 2012; 39(1):119–24.

94. Akizuki M, Sugimura K, Aoki T, et al. Non-invasive screening using ventilatory gas analysis to distinguish between chronic thromboembolic pulmonary hypertension and pulmonary arterial hypertension. Respirology 2020;25(4):427–34.

95. Vicenzi M, Deboeck G, Faoro V, et al. Exercise oscillatory ventilation in heart failure and in pulmonary arterial hypertension. Int J Cardiol 2016;202: 736–40.

96. Jain CC, Borlaug BA. Performance and interpretation of invasive hemodynamic exercise testing. Chest 2020;158(5):2119–29.

97. Lewis GD, Bossone E, Naeije R, et al. Pulmonary vascular hemodynamic response to exercise in cardiopulmonary diseases. Circulation 2013; 128(13):1470–9.

98. Ho JE, Zern EK, Lau ES, et al. Exercise pulmonary hypertension predicts clinical outcomes in patients with dyspnea on effort. J Am Coll Cardiol 2020; 75(1):17–26.

99. Kusunose K, Yamada H, Hotchi J, et al. Prediction of future overt pulmonary hypertension by 6-min walk stress echocardiography in patients with connective tissue disease. J Am Coll Cardiol 2015; 66(4):376–84.

100. Montani D, Girerd B, Jaïs X, et al. Screening for pulmonary arterial hypertension in adults carrying a BMPR2 mutation. Eur Respir J 2021;58(1).

101. Blumberg FC, Arzt M, Lange T, et al. Impact of right ventricular reserve on exercise capacity and survival in patients with pulmonary hypertension. Eur J Heart Fail 2013;15(7):771–5.

102. Eisman AS, Shah RV, Dhakal BP, et al. Pulmonary capillary wedge pressure patterns during exercise predict exercise capacity and incident heart failure. Circulation Heart failure 2018;11(5):e004750.

103. Esfandiari S, Wolsk E, Granton D, et al. Pulmonary arterial wedge pressure at rest and during exercise in healthy adults: a systematic review and meta-analysis. J Card Fail 2019;25(2):114–22.

104. Müller J, Mayer L, Schneider SR, et al. Pulmonary arterial wedge pressure increase during exercise in patients diagnosed with pulmonary arterial or chronic thromboembolic pulmonary hypertension. ERJ open research 2023;9(5):00379–2023.

105. Pieske B, Tschöpe C, de Boer RA, et al. How to diagnose heart failure with preserved ejection fraction: the HFA-PEFF diagnostic algorithm: a consensus recommendation from the Heart Failure Association (HFA) of the European Society of Cardiology (ESC). Eur Heart J 2019;40(40):3297–317.

106. Laveneziana P, Paolo MD, Palange P. The clinical value of cardiopulmonary exercise testing in the modern era. Eur Respir Rev 2021;30(159):200187.

107. Groepenhoff H, Vonk-Noordegraaf A, van de Veerdonk MC, et al. Prognostic relevance of changes in exercise test variables in pulmonary arterial hypertension. PLoS One 2013;8(9):e72013.

108. Hirashiki A, Kondo T, Adachi S, et al. Goal-Oriented Sequential Combination Therapy Evaluated Using Cardiopulmonary Exercise Parameters for the Treatment of Newly Diagnosed Pulmonary Arterial Hypertension - Goal-Oriented Therapy Evaluated by Cardiopulmonary Exercise Testing for Pulmonary Arterial Hypertension (GOOD EYE). Circulation 2019;1(7):303–11.

The Non-invasive Assessment of the Pulmonary Circulation-Right Ventricular Functional Unit
Diagnostic and Prognostic Implications

Federica Giardino, MD[a,b,1], Philipp Douschan, MD, PhD[c,d,e,1],
Stefania Paolillo, MD, PhD[f], Christian Basile, MD[f,g],
Filippo Cademartiri, MD, PhD[h], Francesca Musella, MD, PhD[g,i],
Antonio Cittadini, MD[b,j], Alberto Maria Marra, MD, PhD, FEFIM (hon)[b,*]

KEYWORDS

- Pulmonary hypertension • Right ventricular dysfunction • Non-invasive test
- Cardiopulmonary interactions

KEY POINTS

- Pulmonary circulation-right ventricular functional unit represents a crucial prognostic determinant of several cardiorespiratory diseases.
- Non-invasive techniques allow early diagnosis and tailored therapeutic strategies.
- The development and implementation of new imaging tools may provide key insights into disease-related management.

INTRODUCTION

The pulmonary circulation and the right ventricle (RV) play a pivotal role in the global hemodynamics of human beings, so much so that their close interaction is encapsulated in the concept of a "morpho-functional unit". Historically, research into the RV and its relationship with pulmonary circulation has been overshadowed by studies on its left-sided counterpart. However, recent years have witnessed significant advancements in understanding pulmonary vascular diseases and

[a] Cardiovascular Pathophysiology and Therapeutics (CardioPath) Program, University of Naples Federico II, Via S. Pansini 5, Naples 80131, Italy; [b] Division of Internal Medicine and Metabolism and Rehabilitation, Department of Translational Medical Sciences, University of Naples Federico II, Via S. Pansini 5, Bld.18, 1st Floor, Naples 80131, Italy; [c] Division of Pulmonology, Medical University of Graz, Auenbruggerplatz 15, Graz A-8036, Austria; [d] Division of Pulmonology and Ludwig Boltzmann Institute for Lung Vascular Research, Medical University of Graz, Graz, Austria; [e] Universities of Giessen and Marburg Lung Center (UGMLC), Justus-Liebig-University, Giessen, Germany; [f] Department of Advanced Biomedical Sciences, University of Naples Federico II, Via S. Pansini 5, Building. 2, Naples 80131, Italy; [g] Division of Cardiology, Department of Medicine, Karolinska Institutet, K2 Medicin, Solna, K2 Kardio Lund L Savarese G, Solnavägen 1, Solna, Stockholm 171 77, Sweden; [h] Department of Imaging, Fondazione Monasterio/CNR, Via Giuseppe Moruzzi 1, Pisa 56124, Italy; [i] Cardiology Department, Santa Maria delle Grazie Hospital, Via Domitiana, Pozzuoli, Naples 80078, Italy; [j] Department of Internal Medicine and Clinical Complexity, University of Naples Federico II, Via S. Pansini 5, Building.18, 1st Floor, Naples 80131, Italy
[1] Authors contributed equally.
* Corresponding author.
E-mail address: albertomaria.marra@unina.it

Heart Failure Clin 21 (2025) 63–78
https://doi.org/10.1016/j.hfc.2024.08.004
1551-7136/25/© 2024 Elsevier Inc. All rights are reserved, including those for text and data mining, AI training, and similar technologies.

their impacts on right heart function. Despite progress in therapies for pulmonary arterial hypertension (PAH), clinical improvement and prolonged survival do not consistently result unless accompanied by concurrent enhancements in right ventricular function.[1] Notably, the severity of pulmonary hypertension (PH), as indicated by pulmonary arterial pressure (PAP), does not consistently correlate with symptoms or prognosis, unlike metrics such as RV mass, size, and right atrial pressure, which better reflect functional status and serve as robust predictors of survival.[1,2] The right ventricle displays distinctive anatomic and functional characteristics when compared to the left ventricle (LV). Unlike the LV, the RV is characterized by a larger volume, a thinner free wall (typically ranging between 3 and 5 mm in adults) and a smaller mass.[3] Serving as a crucial cardiac chamber, the RV receives blood from the venous circulation after traversing the right atrium, subsequently propelling it into the pulmonary arteries. The performance of the right ventricle is contingent upon hemodynamic influences, encompassing both preload and afterload, as well as its intrinsic contractility. Variances in pressure, volume or contractility give rise to distinct clinical trajectories and necessitate tailored therapeutic interventions, albeit these conditions often coexist.

While right heart catheterization (RHC) remains the gold standard for diagnosing pulmonary hypertension and gauging disease severity, prognosis, and treatment response, an array of noninvasive tests facilitates the assessment of the pulmonary circulation-right ventricular functional unit (**Fig. 1**; **Table 1**).

SIX-MINUTE WALK TEST

Among the non-invasive techniques for assessing pulmonary hypertension, the six-minute walk test (6MWT) stands out as a simple, safe, well-tolerated, and reproducible tool for evaluating functional exercise capacity of patients. It allows quantification of moderate-to-severe impairment resulting from various pulmonary diseases, while also being sensitive to alterations seen in conditions such as cardiovascular disease, frailty, sarcopenia, and cancer.[4] The 6MWT does not demand a high level of expertise from healthcare staff or complex equipment, making it easily implementable in clinical settings. The test involves measuring the distance (6MWD) a patient can cover in 6 minutes while walking on a straight, level surface, as outlined in the latest American Thoracic Society guidelines.[5] Prior to beginning the 6MWT, vital signs at rest (including blood

pressure, heart rate, and oxygen saturation) are measured using a sphygmomanometer and pulse oximeter. Additionally, patients rate their perception of dyspnea on the Borg scale, selecting a number from 0 (indicating absence of dyspnea) to 10 (representing maximal sustainable dyspnea). During the test, staff does not accompany the patients along the route, nor influence their walking speed.

In addition to assessing exercise capacity, the 6MWT provides insight into potential symptoms that arise during the test, helps assess response to treatment, and allows for the evaluation of patients' prognosis across various cardiopulmonary conditions.[6] Indeed, both the absolute 6MWD and changes in 6MWD serve as predictors of morbidity and mortality in conditions such as chronic obstructive pulmonary disease (COPD), pulmonary arterial hypertension (PAH), idiopathic pulmonary fibrosis (IPF), and among patients awaiting lung transplants.[4,7] Nishiyama and colleagues[8] conducted a study in patients affected by interstitial lung disease, aiming to correlate 6MWT outcomes (6MWD, desaturation, and symptoms) with measurements obtained from pulmonary function tests and right heart catheterization. Their findings revealed that percent predicted forced vital capacity (FVC) and percent predicted diffusing capacity of the lungs for carbon monoxide (DLco) independently predicted 6MWD, while the latter parameter, along with pulmonary vascular resistance (PVR), were independent predictors of oxygen saturation at the end of the 6MWT. The percent predicted DLco independently predicted severity of dyspnea at the end of the test.[8]

Furthermore, the 6MWT is employed to assess the functional capacity of patients with heart failure (HF), aiding in the measurement of exercise capacity and response to therapy. This test effectively quantifies exercise intolerance due to HF, with improvements in functional capacity suggesting positive responses to therapies including medication adjustments or cardiac rehabilitation programs.[9]

By measuring exercise tolerance, this tool reflects the impact of PH on daily activities due to increased PVR and impaired cardiac output, as well as disease progression. A shorter 6MWD during the 6MWT may indicate worsening symptoms and a decline in functional status, thus leading to a poor prognosis.[10] In a study by Paciocco and colleagues,[11] it was highlighted that in patients with untreated primary pulmonary hypertension, a distance of ≤300 m increased mortality risk by 2.4, while a difference in oxygen saturation (delta SaO2) ≥10% increased mortality risk by 2.9.

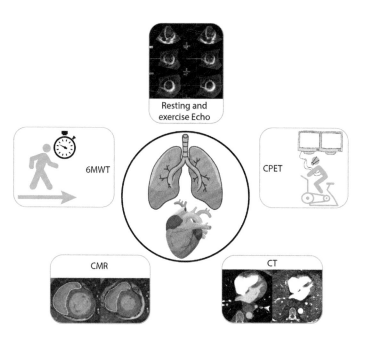

Oxygen saturation at peak distance, delta SaO2, and pulmonary vascular resistance were also related to mortality.[11] The exercise limitation assessed through a reduced distance during the 6MWT serves as an excellent predictor of death in PAH. Specifically, a greater 6MWD in patients with idiopathic, familial, and anorexigen-associated PAH correlates positively with survival.[12] Benza and colleagues[13] demonstrated that a 6MWD ≥440 m was associated with increased 1-year survival in PAH patients, while Souza and colleagues[14] highlighted that PAH patients at Month 6 of the SERAPHIN trial (patients randomized to placebo or macitentan) who were able to walk more than 400 m during the 6MWT had a better long-term prognosis, in terms of PAH-related death or hospitalization or all-cause death.

Thus, the 6MWT not only evaluates physical performance but also reflects the overall impact of PH on patients' quality of life.[15] Furthermore, it enables physicians to tailor interventions and optimize care plans based on individual patient needs.

In conclusion, the 6MWT provides insights into the impact of PH and HF on patients' daily lives, aiding healthcare providers in making informed decisions about treatment strategies and monitoring the effectiveness of interventions. Regular use of this tool contributes to a holistic approach to patient care, emphasizing the importance of addressing both the physiologic and functional aspects of these cardiovascular conditions.

ECHOCARDIOGRAPHY AT REST

Transthoracic Doppler Echocardiography (TDE) is a widely used, low-cost, easy-to-perform exam and first-line diagnostic tool for non-invasive evaluation of pulmonary circulation-right ventricular unit (**Fig. 2**). In this field of application, it can be helpful for some main purposes: (1) screening of patients with suspected PH; (2) generating hypotheses about the possible etiology of PH; (3) helping to identify patients for whom invasive hemodynamic evaluation by right heart catheterization is indicated; (4) investigating the hemodynamic consequences of PH on the right heart-pulmonary circulation unit.

TDE allows estimation of right ventricular systolic pressure (RVSP) by analyzing the peak tricuspid regurgitation velocity (peak TRV or Vmax) with continuous Doppler. The accuracy of TDE in estimating pulmonary circulation pressures was previously analyzed in 1984 by Yock and colleagues,[16] who demonstrated a good correlation (r = .93) between non-invasive echocardiographic estimation and invasive evaluation by heart catheterization.

The systolic pressure gradient between the right ventricle and right atrium (delta-P) is estimated by the modified Bernoulli equation (delta-P = $4 \cdot Vmax^2$). RVSP can be obtained by adding the hypothetical value of right atrium pressure (RAP), which is estimated by the dimension and collapsibility of the inferior vena cava.[17] In the absence of a pressure gradient across the pulmonary valve

Table 1
Main advantages and drawbacks of the most used non-invasive techniques for the assessment of the right ventricular and pulmonary circulation unit

Technique	Advantages	Drawbacks	Notes
Six-Minute Walk Test (6MWT)	• Easy to perform • Reproducible • Fast and well-tolerated • Inexpensive • No high-level expertise required • Simple equipment	• Sensitive to different pathologic alterations • No information on mechanisms of exercise limitation	• Allows quantification of moderate-to-severe impairment of pulmonary diseases. • Predicts morbidity and mortality in PAH, IPF, COPD and patients awaiting lung transplant.
Transthoracic Doppler Echocardiography (TDE)	• Highly available • Affordable • No radiation exposure • Anatomic and functional assessment of the heart • Portable	• Operator dependence • Inadequate imaging in poor acoustic windows • No evaluation of lung • No direct evaluation of pressures in pulmonary circulation	• Helpful for screening of patients with suspected PH and generating hypotheses about PH etiology. • Good correlation with RHC for assessing pressures of pulmonary circulation. • Evaluations under stress are possible.
Computed Tomography (CT)	• Superior spatial and contrast resolution • Unlimited imaging window • Evaluation of both heart and lung anatomy	• Elevated radiation exposure • Utilization of iodinated contrast agents • Lack of functional evaluation • Higher cost	• Using Photon Counting CT (PCCT) is routinely feasible to perform tissue characterization imaging as CMR. • Exploiting CFD simulations more advanced information on flow dynamics are available.
CardioPulmonary Exercise Test (CPET)	• No radiation exposure • Assessment of functional status and RV function • Details on etiology of exercise limitation	• Limited availability • Requires high expertise • Requires clinically stable and collaborative patients	• Provides insights into the cardiovascular respiratory metabolic and muscular responses in physical exertion. • Prognostic tool for PAH patient.
Cardiac Magnetic Resonance (CMR)	• High spatial and temporal resolution • Reproducibility • Unlimited imaging window • No radiation exposure	• Impractical for patients with metal implants or incompatible electronic devices • Breath-holding requirement • Extended scan duration • Substantially increased expenses	• Gold standard for RV and LV assessment. • CMR-derived RV strain correlates with RV-arterial uncoupling and diastolic RV stiffness.

Abbreviations: CFD, computational fluid dynamics; COPD, chronic obstructive pulmonary disease; IPF, idiopathic pulmonary fibrosis; LV, left ventricle; PAH, pulmonary arterial hypertension; PH, pulmonary hypertension; RHC, right heart catheterization; RV, right ventricle.

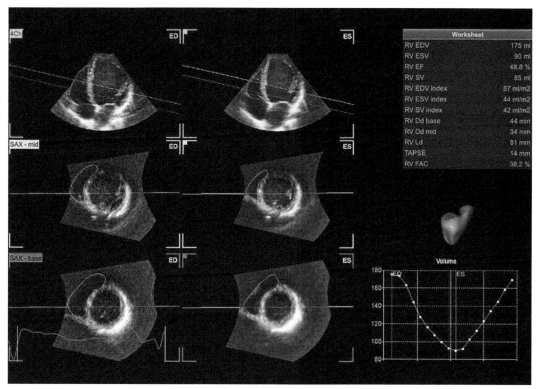

Worksheet	
RV EDV	175 ml
RV ESV	90 ml
RV EF	48.8 %
RV SV	85 ml
RV EDV index	87 ml/m2
RV ESV index	44 ml/m2
RV SV index	42 ml/m2
RV Dd base	44 mm
RV Dd mid	34 mm
RV Ld	81 mm
TAPSE	14 mm
RV FAC	38.2 %

Fig. 2. Resting echocardiographic parameters for the assessment of the right ventricular dimension and function in a patient with a mildly impaired right ventricular contractile function. In the lower right-hand corner of the figure, the graph shows the difference in volume of the right ventricle between end-diastole (ED; maximum volume) and end-systole (ES; minimum volume), related to its ability to take blood during diastole and pump it out during systole. 4Ch, apical four-chamber view; ED, end-diastole; ES, end-systole; RV Dd base, right ventricular basal diameter at end-diastole; RV Dd mid, right ventricular mid-level diameter at end-diastole; RV EDV, right ventricular end-diastolic volume; RV EF, right ventricular ejection fraction; RV ESV, right ventricular end-systolic volume; RV FAC, right ventricular fractional area change; RV Ld, right ventricular longitudinal diameter at end-diastole; RV SV, right ventricular stroke volume; SAX-base, parasternal short axis view at base-ventricular level; SAX-mid, parasternal short axis view at mid-ventricular level; TAPSE, tricuspid annular plane systolic excursion.

or right ventricle outflow tract (RVOT), the RVSP equals systolic pulmonary artery pressure (sPAP).

Considering the high variability in the estimation of RAP, current ESC PH Guidelines[18] recommend the use of the peak TRV velocity value to assess the probability of PH (low, intermediate, or high). If the peak TRV is < 2.8 m/sec PH is unlikely, while a peak TRV > 3.4 m/sec suggests high probability of PH. When peak TRV is between 2.8 and 3.4 m/sec, the absence or presence of other "echo-PH signs" correlates, respectively, with intermediate or high probability of PH.[18]

TDE is also useful in helping generating hypotheses about PH etiology, and discriminating between "pre-capillary PH" and "post-capillary PH" echocardiographic patterns.[19]

TDE is helpful in identifying signs of post-capillary PH (WHO Group 2 PH due to left heart disease), which is the most common form of

PH.[18] Etiologies of post-capillary PH detectable by TDE include mitral or aortic valvular disease, chronic ischemic myocardial disease, systolic and/or diastolic LV dysfunction, LV dilatation and LV hypertrophy.

Pre-capillary PH is suspected when echocardiographic features ("echo-PH signs") are detected, including RV and/or RA dilatation, RV hypertrophy, tricuspid regurgitation and TR jet velocity, notched pulsed wave-Doppler (PW-Doppler) in the RVOT, inferior vena cava dilatation, or evidence of right ventricular pressure overload including distortion of LV geometry with displacement of the interventricular septum during end-systole (a "D-shape" of LV).[19] It is important to note that discrimination between "pre-capillary" or "post-capillary PH" necessarily requires diagnostic confirmation by RHC.

The pathophysiological phenomenon that leads to PH development is a progressive pulmonary vascular remodeling resulting in increased pulmonary vascular resistance leading to a subsequent raise in RV pressure. At the early stages of PH, the RV adapts to the increased arterial load by enhancing contractility and wall thickness ("coupling"). Progressive RV dilatation and/or dysfunction ("uncoupling") occurs at the end-stage of the disease, which is ultimately characterized by right heart failure and high mortality.[20]

Recently, the ratio between tricuspid annular plane systolic excursion (TAPSE) and the sPAP estimated has been validated as an echocardiographic parameter capable of describing the RV–Arterial Coupling "strength".

The prognostic role of "TAPSE/sPAP ratio" in heart failure was first described by Guazzi and colleagues[21] Recent studies[22,23] have demonstrated that TAPSE/sPAP ratio is also an independent predictor of mortality in PH, and has been validated as a non-invasive tool for risk stratification in PH patients.

EXERCISE ECHOCARDIOGRAPHY

Pulmonary exercise hemodynamics are of increasing interest in the functional assessment of the right heart and pulmonary circulation. Most recently, it has been shown that pathologic pulmonary exercise hemodynamics are characteristics of early stages of pulmonary vascular disease (PVD).[24,25] Exercise parameters have been associated with poor prognosis in patients at risk for PH, and there is increasing evidence for their additive predictive value, as compared to resting hemodynamics, in patients with early pulmonary vascular disease (PVD).[26,27] As a result, the term "exercise pulmonary hypertension" (EPH) has been reintroduced into international guidelines for the diagnosis and treatment of PH.[18] EPH is currently defined by a mean pulmonary arterial pressure to cardiac output (mPAP/CO) slope > 3 mm Hg/L/min, assessed by invasive exercise right heart catheterization. However, invasive assessment of pulmonary exercise hemodynamics is technically challenging, and not readily available at all centers. Non-invasive approaches using exercise echocardiography have been established and proposed in several clinical studies.[28–30]

Protocols using physical exercise testing on a bicycle ergometer in a semi-supine position combined with echocardiography are most widely used for the investigation of the right pulmonary circulation-right ventricular unit.[28] By using an incremental stepwise increase of workload, RV functional parameters of interest and RV afterload can be assessed at each level of exercise. The measurement of tricuspid regurgitation velocity by continuous wave-Doppler (CW-Doppler) and estimates of sPAP and mPAP based on the TRV have been implemented in stress echocardiography protocols for a long time. A steep increase of PAP estimates during stress testing may serve as a first indication of early pulmonary vascular disease. Dynamic changes in ventricular afterload during physical exercise testing always need to be interpreted together with cardiac output, as pulmonary arterial pressure during exercise is highly dependent on workload and blood flow. Cardiac output can be non-invasively determined using the PW-Doppler derived velocity time integral (VTI) measured in either the RVOT or the left ventricular outflow tract (LVOT). It is important to acknowledge that both TRV-derived PAP and VTI-derived CO are estimates of cardiopulmonary hemodynamics, and normative values based on exercise echocardiography may differ significantly from established cut-offs based on invasive exercise RHC data. A recent large, multi-center study identified clinically relevant differences in mPAP/CO slopes based on exercise echocardiographic measurements from athletes, controls, and patients at risk for PVD.[29] Interestingly, pooled data analysis from athletes and controls revealed an upper limit of normal close to the established invasive mPAP/CO-slope cut-off for defining EPH. The upper limit of the exercise-echocardiography derived mPAP/CO-slopes in healthy subjects was found to be 3.5 mm Hg/L/min, underlining the reliability of exercise echocardiography for the evaluation of pulmonary exercise hemodynamics.[29] Additional parameters reflecting RV function that have been implemented in exercise-echocardiography protocols include TAPSE, S' wave, RV-Strain, 3D ejection fraction (3D-EF) and fractional area change (FAC).[28,30] The TAPSE/sPAP ratio has recently been validated as reliable non-invasive surrogate for right ventricular-pulmonary artery coupling at rest.[23] It is strongly correlated with pulmonary exercise hemodynamics and may serve as additional marker for contractile reserve during non-invasive stress testing.[31] Reported normal ranges of TAPSE/sPAP-ratio during peak exercise are 0.5–1.5 mm/mm Hg.[29]

Impaired exercise performance and abnormal changes in pulmonary hemodynamics during exercise are typical features of early PVD, and they may serve as valuable tools in the screening for PVD. Several screening studies focusing on patients at risk for pulmonary arterial hypertension have been undertaken. These included patients with risk factors for hereditary PAH, chronic thromboembolic disease, scleroderma, and chronic liver disease.[32–35]

Like invasive pulmonary exercise hemodynamics, non-invasive exercise hemodynamics have been shown to be robust predictors of outcome. In addition to their prognostic value in patients with early PVD, their ability to investigate contractile reserve in patients with advanced PH may serve as future prognosticator in the risk assessment of patients with PH. In patients at risk for or diagnosed with PH, a non-invasive mPAP/CO slope > 5 mm Hg/L/min was recently found as predictor of all-cause mortality.[29]

The evaluation of the pulmonary circulation-right ventricular functional unit during exercise has expaned our understanding of the interaction between the right heart and the pulmonary circulation. We are currently observing the dawn of a new era aimed at more deeply phenotyping pulmonary vascular and right ventricular pathologies. Due to its availability, non-invasive approach, and strong ability to display different aspects of the RV function and anatomy, exercise echocardiography will continue to play an important role in the diagnosis and management of pulmonary vascular disease.

CARDIOPULMONARY EXERCISE TEST

The Cardiopulmonary Exercise Test (CPET) is another highly effective, non-invasive tool for evaluating the role of pulmonary circulation-right ventricular (dys-)function in exercise limitation.[36] By analyzing functional capacity in various settings, CPET provides valuable insights into the cardiovascular, respiratory, metabolic, and muscular responses that occur during physical exertion. This allows for the identification of potential impairments affecting exercise limitation, particularly those related to pulmonary circulation-right ventricular function.[37]

During exercise, healthy individuals increase ventilation while decreasing the ratio of 'functional' dead space to tidal volume (Vd/Vt), resulting in an improved efficacy of the ventilation/perfusion (V/Q) match.[38] However, in clinical conditions such as pulmonary embolism and pulmonary hypertension, ventilation increases but pulmonary vascular bed recruitment decreases, leading to ineffective perfusion and a rise in mean V/Q and functional Vd/Vt. This can cause dyspnea during exercise due to compromised gas exchange efficiency. To diagnose and manage these patients effectively, the slope of the relationship between minute ventilation and carbon dioxide production (VE/VCO2 slope) measured by CPET can be critical. Patients with PH display a significant increase in VE/VCO2 slope due to inefficient ventilation during exercise.[39] The increase in functional Vd/Vt and ventilation leads to a decrease in end-tidal pressure of carbon dioxide (PETCO2) both at rest and during exercise.

The proper function of the right ventricle is crucial for maintaining an adequate increase in stroke volume during physical activity, and right ventricular dysfunction can lead to an inability of cardiac output to increase during exercise. This can cause a lack of oxygen delivery during exercise, which can lead to lactic acidosis, even at low work rates. Lactic acidosis results in increased $H+$ concentrations and an increase in carbon dioxide (CO_2) produced by HCO_3 buffering. These factors can contribute to the stimulation of the ventilatory drive and the sensation of dyspnea during physical activity.[40] All these components can be assessed using CPET, which can reveal a reduction in peak oxygen consumption (Vo_2 peak), Vo_2 at the anaerobic threshold, Vo_2/work relationship, and oxygen pulse as indirect indexes of impaired cardiac output.

During exercise, a drop in oxygen saturation of at least 3% without a rise in $Paco_2$, known as desaturation, is a significant indicator of pulmonary vascular exercise limitation. This behavior is often observed in patients with moderate forms of pulmonary circulation-right ventricular dysfunction, particularly those with at least moderate pulmonary hypertension. The degree of reduction is directly proportional to the severity of the disease.[41]

In addition to established CPET parameters, emerging variables such as the oxygen uptake efficiency (OUE) plateau and OUE slope are being explored to indicate ventilatory inefficiency during exercise in PH patients. Research by Tan and colleagues[42] and Zhao and colleagues[43] has shown lower OUE slope and OUE plateau values in PH patients, indicating their potential diagnostic relevance. However, further research and data are needed to validate and confirm these initial findings.

Therefore, CPET can be recommended for clinically stable patients with conditions affecting pulmonary circulation who can undergo exercise testing (**Table 2**). It can aid in the diagnosis of conditions contributing to exercise limitation, assess functional status, assess disease severity, and provide prognostic information[44] (**Fig. 3**). Despite its potential benefits, limited availability outside third-level centers means its use is still infrequent in these patients.

COMPUTED TOMOGRAPHY

Among cardiovascular imaging techniques, Computed Tomography (CT) has rapidly evolved over the past 25 years.[45–49] Moreover, it has

Table 2
Typical cardiopulmonary exercise testing parameters in patients with conditions affecting the pulmonary circulation

Parameters	PH
Peak Vo_2	Reduced
Vo_2 at AT	Reduced
Vo_2/WR	Reduced
O_2 pulse	Reduced
Peak VE	Reduced
Breathing reserve	Normal
VE/VCO$_2$ slope	Increased
VE/VCO$_2$ at AT	Increased
PETCO$_2$	Reduced
SaO$_2$	Reduced

Abbreviations: AT, anaerobic threshold; O2, oxygen; Peak VE, peak minute ventilation; Peak Vo2, peak oxygen uptake; PETCO2, end-tidal pressure of carbon dioxide; PH, pulmonary hypertension; SaO2, oxygen saturation; VCO2, carbon dioxide production; WR, work rate.

been enhanced by Photon Counting CT (PCCT) generation.[50–56]

CT Angiography (CTA) is well established for non-invasive pulmonary embolism (PE) assessment, but its routine use for evaluating the pulmonary circulation-RV function unit has not been extensively explored.[57–61] ECG synchronization techniques since 1999 have advanced Cardiac CT (CCT).[45–49] However, the potential of this technology for detailed assessment of the pulmonary circulation-RV function unit has been quite limited. Initial limitations included: (1) CT's inability to measure flow; (2) previous lack of the most advanced ECG synchronization techniques, which have been available for echocardiography and magnetic resonance (MR) for quite some time; and (3) the relatively high radiation doses required in the early phases of its development.

Nevertheless, the anatomic and morphologic diagnostic capabilities of CT, CTA, and CCT are now unrivaled, compared to non-invasive and invasive diagnostic tools. Currently, chest CT plays a critical role role in angiographic and morphologic assessments due to its panoramic approach, high-resolution and detailed unrestricted three-dimensional capabilities. With the pairing of ECG-gating/triggering techniques (CCT), detailed assessments at the level of the coronary arteries, all cardiac chambers, and great thoracic vessels are routinely available.

However, there are several aspects of the diagnostic potential of CT that are underappreciated.

CCT can play the same role as CMR and echocardiography in providing reference standards for cardiac chamber functional and volumetric

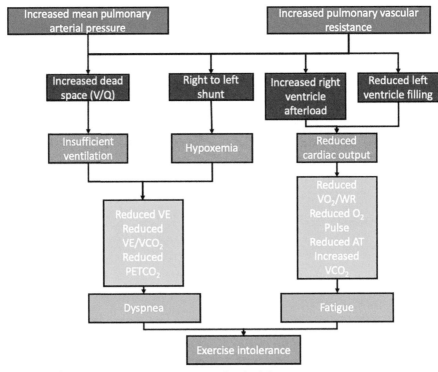

Fig. 3. How Cardiopulmonary exercise test connects pathophysiology to symptoms.

assessment.[62,63] Besides the fact that CCT provides near-perfect panoramic 3D and 4D representation and quantification of cardiac chambers with temporal resolution, it has no anatomic restrictions, can also overcome issues related to devices that are not compatible with (or are MR-conditional) and it is feasible for patients to undergo imaging even in non-fully cooperative clinical conditions. Finally, CT provides all the anatomic context possible of the structures around the pulmonary circulation–right ventricular function unit; particularly the lung parenchyma and intra-parenchymal vascularization (both arterial and venous).

CT's clinical applications include.

- Diagnosis of pulmonary embolism, via CT pulmonary angiography (CTPA).
- Pulmonary artery assessment, providing detailed images of the pulmonary arteries, helping to evaluate their size, shape, and patency. This is important for identifying conditions such as pulmonary hypertension, pulmonary artery stenosis, or aneurysms.
- Diagnosis of congenital heart diseases: it helps visualize abnormalities such as ventricular septal defects, atrial septal defects, and other structural anomalies.
- Diagnosis of Chronic Thromboembolic Pulmonary Hypertension (CTEPH), allowing the identification of the location and extent of chronic thromboembolic disease.
- Assessment of the Right Ventricular Dysfunction/Overload, providing information about the size of the right ventricle.
- Diagnosis of cardiac anomalies.
- Preoperative Planning.

In the last 2 years we have witnessed the introduction of the latest generation of CT technology allowing the reduction in the necessary radiation dose as compared to all previous generation of CT technologies. In the light of this quantum technological leap, we will have to reframe our current and future expectations from the diagnostic relevance of PCCT in every field including pulmonary circulation–right ventricular function unit (**Figs. 4 and 5**). The concurrent development of artificial intelligence (AI)/Deep learning assisted algorithms allows extensive implementation of CCT as a primary diagnostic tool in clinical practice.

State-of-the-art CT technology, and especially PCCT, offers high spatial resolution and spectral capabilities, allowing routine clinical assessments of.

- LV/RV volumes, function, myocardial mass, wall thickness, wall motion, longitudinal and radial strain.

- Left atrium (LA)/right atrium (RA) volumes, function and strain.
- Intra-cavitary masses.
- Cardiac valves.
- Entire morphology and patency of pulmonary artery and distal pulmonary artery branches beyond sub-segmental arteries (**Fig. 6**).
- Pulmonary/lung spectral perfusion with Dual Energy geometry or with full spectral capabilities with PCCT.

Using PCCT it is routinely feasible to perform tissue characterization imaging as in CMR; for instance, it is possible to evaluate areas of delayed arterial perfusion (ie, perfusion defects acute and chronic) and delayed contrast enhancement representing fibrotic degeneration or previous ischemic myocardial wall damage.

More advanced investigational evaluations of flow can be performed using Computational Fluid Dynamics (CFD) delivering a 4D-flow assessment of cardiac chambers and great thoracic vessels, but at the moment this kind of analyses are performed only in advanced imaging research labs.

The main limitation of CT/CCT beyond consolidated CTA applications for acute and chronic thrombo-embolic disease is related to the lack of large validation and/or technology comparison studies available to refer to for the actual clinical implementation. In addition, there is still scarce availability of advanced state-of-the-art CT equipment and technical competence of dedicated personnel for clinical applications that are not mainstream.

In a recent study, the diagnostic accuracy of CT pulmonary angiography was evaluated in patients suspected of having pulmonary hypertension.[64] The study identified models that enabled stratification of these patients based on their mortality risk and patients who were determined not to have PH on CT scans showed an excellent prognosis.[64]

Additionally, already for many years, CT has been considered for evaluating RV and LV morphology and function in patient affected by primary pulmonary hypertension, both at rest and under stress.[65] In recent years, there has been a rapid development in stress CT to assess perfusion abnormalities and myocardial tissue.[66] However, high radiation exposure, motion artifacts and lack protocol uniformity remain the primary limitations to a broader clinical use of stress CT.[66]

CARDIAC MAGNETIC RESONANCE

Ultrasound imaging of the RV presents numerous challenges due to its anatomic location behind the sternum, its intricate shape, and the presence

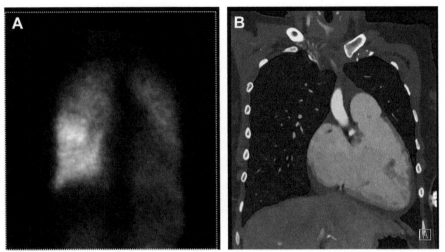

Fig. 4. Ventilation/Perfusion Lung Scintigraphy and Spectral Cardiac/Coronary/Thoracic PCCT example of normal pulmonary perfusion in a Grown-Up Congenital Heart Disease (GUCH) patient. The figure shows a Grown-Up Congenital Heart Disease (GUCH) patient studied with Ventilation/Perfusion Lung Scintigraphy (*A*) and Spectral Cardiac/Coronary/Thoracic PCCT (*B*) with VNC + overlay of iodine map. The lung perfusion is normal and there is a dilated RV. The scan was performed on a commercial whole-body Dual Source Photon Counting CT scanner (NAEOTOM Alpha, Siemens Healthineers) with 0.2/0.4 mm slice thickness, 0.1/0.2 mm reconstruction increment, FOV 200 to 250 mm, resolution matrix of 512x512/1024x1024 pixels on the source axial reconstructions with a kernel filtering of Bv48 to 60 (vascular kernel medium-sharp) and with maximum intensity of Quantum Iterative Reconstruction (QIR 4); the scan is performed with retrospective ECG gating with tube current modulation. The displayed spatial resolution is 0.1/0.20 mm. PCCT, Photon Counting CT; RV, Right Ventricle; VNC, Virtual Non-Contrast.

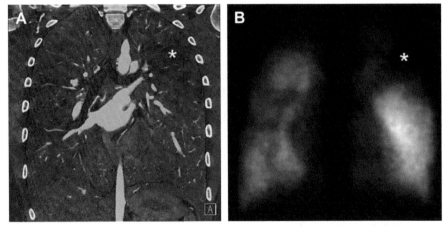

Fig. 5. Spectral Cardiac/Coronary PCCT and Ventilation/Perfusion Lung Scintigraphy in a patient with mild Pulmonary Hypertension. The figure shows a patient with Pulmonary Hypertension studied with Spectral Cardiac/Coronary/Thoracic PCCT (*A*; VNC + overlay of iodine map) and Ventilation/Perfusion Lung Scintigraphy (*B*). The lung perfusion is abnormal with sharp segmental defect on the left upper lobe (*in A and B). The scan was performed on a commercial whole-body Dual Source Photon Counting CT scanner (NAEOTOM Alpha, Siemens Healthineers) with 0.2/0.4 mm slice thickness, 0.1/0.2 mm reconstruction increment, FOV 200 to 250 mm, resolution matrix of 512x512/1024x1024 pixels on the source axial reconstructions with a kernel filtering of Bv48 to 60 (vascular kernel medium-sharp) and with maximum intensity of Quantum Iterative Reconstruction (QIR 4); the scan is performed with retrospective ECG gating with tube current modulation. The displayed spatial resolution is 0.1/0.20 mm. PCCT, Photon Counting CT; VNC, Virtual Non-Contrast.

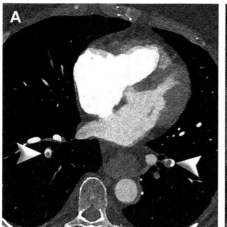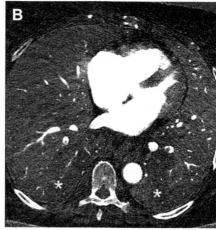

Fig. 6. Spectral Cardiac/Coronary/Thoracic PCCT example of sub-acute pulmonary embolism. The figure shows a patient with Pulmonary Hypertension studied with Spectral Cardiac/Coronary/Thoracic PCCT (*A*: CT Angiography with Monochromatic + at 40 KeV; *B*: Spectral Iodine image). There are perfusion defects in the lobar segmental branches for the lower lobes bilaterally (*A; arrowheads*); in the Spectral Iodine image there are clear perfusion defects in the medial portions of lower lobes bilaterally (*in *B*). The scan was performed on a commercial whole-body Dual Source Photon Counting CT scanner (NAEOTOM Alpha, Siemens Healthineers) with 0.2/0.4 mm slice thickness, 0.1/0.2 mm reconstruction increment, FOV 200 to 250 mm, resolution matrix of 512x512/1024x1024 pixels on the source axial reconstructions with a kernel filtering of Bv48 to 60 (vascular kernel medium-sharp) and with maximum intensity of Quantum Iterative Reconstruction (QIR 4); the scan is performed with retrospective ECG gating with tube current modulation. The displayed spatial resolution is 0.1/0.20 mm. PCCT, Photon Counting CT.

of multiple trabeculations. These factors can impede the clarity and accuracy of ultrasound images when studying the RV structure and mechanics. On the contrary, cardiac magnetic resonance imaging (CMR) offers distinctive advantages in assessing the right chambers and is recommended as the gold standard for quantifying RV size, mass, and function.[67,68] The most commonly utilized cine sequences in CMR for RV assessment are the segmented steady-state free precession (SSFP). These sequences, acquired during breath-holding and ECG-gating, provide high spatial and temporal resolution, exceptional reproducibility, and intrinsic contrast, making them well-suited for comprehensive RV analysis.[69] RV volume and mass can be accurately quantified using Simpson's method, involving tracing the RV endocardial border across multiple short-axis slices and computing the total volume through summation (**Fig. 7**). Long axis planes (horizontal long axis–HLA, right ventricle outflow tract–RVOT, and RV 2-chamber views) can be interrogated to assess global and regional wall motion abnormalities (normokinesis, hypokinesis, akinesis, and dyskinesis), while transaxial cine stack images are pivotal for evaluating RV free wall profile and function (**Fig. 8**). A significant advantage of SSFP cine sequences is their compatibility with feature tracking (FT) techniques, akin to

echocardiographic speckle tracking. FT entails identifying and tracking specific points of interest within the myocardium, facilitating the quantification of myocardial strain and deformation. By tracking subendocardial and subepicardial points of interest, FT offers valuable insights into myocardial mechanics and function, enhancing the comprehensive assessment of the RV. Late Gadolinium Enhancement (LGE) sequences, acquired 10 to 20 minutes after contrast agent administration, are routinely utilized in CMR to identify diseased myocardium corresponding to zones of myocyte necrosis or myocardial fibrosis, as demonstrated by comparison with histopathology.[70]

The ability to non-invasively and reproducibly assess RV structure and mechanics is crucial due to the well-recognized prognostic value in various pathologic conditions, particularly in PH patients. Multiple studies underscore RV function as a primary predictor of long-term outcomes, irrespective of PH etiology.[71] In a recent meta-analysis involving 1,938 participants with PAH, CMR-derived parameters including RV ejection fraction and indexed volumes were identified as predictors not only of outcomes but also of clinical worsening.[72] Routinely evaluating RV volume and mass during follow-up is imperative, as both parameters are considered treatment targets. Notably, patients with low RV volume and mass

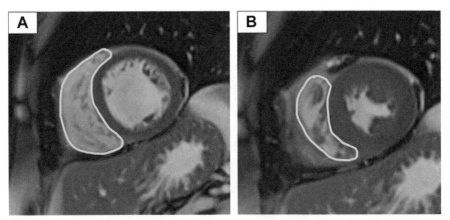

Fig. 7. Segmented steady-state free precession (SSFP) short-axis views (*A* = diastole; *B* = systole).

on CMR assessment exhibit lower mortality rates than those with high RV volume and low RV mass, likely due to maladaptation to the increased RV afterload.[73] Systematically evaluating RV strain in PH using CMR-FT is both feasible and reproducible, with RV strain measures correlating with disease severity and clinical deterioration. Specifically, RV global circumferential strain rate (GCSR) remains associated with outcomes even after adjustment for other prognostic predictors in PH.[74] Moreover, CMR-derived RV strain significantly correlates with RV-arterial uncoupling and diastolic RV stiffness as measured via right heart catheterization.[75]

Regarding fibrosis, LGE is commonly observed in patients with PH, often localized at the level of the RV insertion points alone or concurrent with interventricular septum involvement (**Fig. 9**). While the presence of LGE holds diagnostic significance and is typically linked with greater RV dilation, it is not associated with an additional increase in mortality.[76]

Moreover, exercise CMR provides a wide range of diagnostic opportunities, including the assessment of cardiac chamber dimensions and function, stress perfusion imaging, flow studies, and tissue characterization.[77] To address the limitation of breath-held acquisition methods during stress CMR, the real-time cine imaging allows for free-breathing during exercise. In addition to its established role in detecting coronary artery disease and providing prognostic data, exercise CMR has also developed for managing congenital heart disease and congestive heart failure.[77] It serves as a crucial tool for characterizing the pulmonary circulation and right ventricular functional unit, helping to identify abnormal pulmonary vascular function that may not be apparent at rest.[77]

In conclusion, CMR is a key imaging test to thoroughly study the RV sections, and it is mandatory in profiling PH patients as the study of the right heart is crucial for diagnosis, prognostication, clinical follow-up, and evaluation of response to treatment.

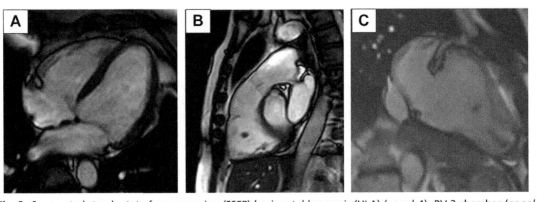

Fig. 8. Segmented steady-state free precession (SSFP) horizontal long axis (HLA) (*panel A*), RV 2-chamber (*panel B*), and right ventricle outflow tract (RVOT) views (*panel C*).

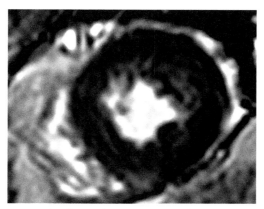

Fig. 9. Late gadolinium enhancement (LGE) at right ventricle insertion points.

SUMMARY

In recent decades, increasing emphasis has been placed on the coupling between the right ventricle and pulmonary artery. Significant strides have been made in the treatment of pulmonary hypertension, and greater attention has been directed toward early diagnosis of this condition. Consequently, noninvasive examinations, such as the 6-min walk test, resting and stress echocardiography, cardiopulmonary exercise test, cardiac CT, and CMR, have assumed a pivotal role in exploring the anatomy and function of the right ventricle-pulmonary circulation unit. While the diagnosis of pulmonary hypertension relies on invasive measurements during right heart catheterization, these noninvasive techniques, apart from being valuable in early detection of structural and/or functional abnormalities of the right ventricle-pulmonary circulation unit, aid in patient management and prognostic stratification. Moreover, advancements in modern technologies have greatly enhanced the performance of these methods, thereby improving their accuracy.

CLINICS CARE POINTS

- Resting and stress echocardiography, cardiopulmonary exercise testing, computed tomography, and cardiac magnetic resonance allow the non-invasive characterization of the pulmonary circulation-right ventricular unit both morphologically and functionally.

- The echocardiographic TAPSE/sPAP ratio is an independent predictor of mortality in PH patients and has been validated as a non-invasive tool for risk stratification in PH patients.

- The evaluation of the pulmonary circulation-right ventricular functional unit during exercise has increased the understanding of the interaction between the right heart and the pulmonary circulation.

- CPET can aid in the diagnosis of conditions contributing to exercise limitation, in the assessment of functional status and disease severity, and in providing prognostic information.

ACKNOWLEDGMENTS

Dr F. Giardino received research grant by the Cardiovascular Pathophysiology and Therapeutics (CardioPath) program from the University of Naples Federico II, Italy. The Authors thank Alessandra Schiavo, Rodolfo Citro and Erica Maffei for outstanding contribution.

DISCLOSURE

The authors declare that they have no conflict of interest.

REFERENCES

1. Champion HC, Michelakis ED, Hassoun PM. Comprehensive invasive and noninvasive approach to the right ventricle-pulmonary circulation unit: state of the art and clinical and research implications. Circulation 2009;120(11):992–1007.
2. Voelkel NF, Quaife RA, Leinwand LA, et al. Right ventricular function and failure: report of a National Heart, Lung, and Blood Institute working group on cellular and molecular mechanisms of right heart failure. Circulation 2006;114(17):1883–91.
3. Sanz J, Sánchez-Quintana D, Bossone E, et al. Anatomy, function, and dysfunction of the right ventricle: JACC state-of-the-art review. J Am Coll Cardiol 2019;73(12):1463–82.
4. Agarwala P, Salzman SH. Six-minute walk test: clinical role, technique, coding, and reimbursement. Chest 2020;157(3):603–11.
5. ATS Committee on Proficiency Standards for Clinical Pulmonary Function Laboratories. ATS statement: guidelines

for the six-minute walk test. Am J Respir Crit Care Med 2002;166(1):111–7.

6. Rasekaba T, Lee AL, Naughton MT, et al. The six-minute walk test: a useful metric for the cardiopulmonary patient. Intern Med J 2009;39(8):495–501.

7. Heresi GA, Dweik RA. Strengths and limitations of the six-minute-walk test: a model biomarker study in idiopathic pulmonary fibrosis. Am J Respir Crit Care Med 2011;183(9):1122–4.

8. Nishiyama O, Yamazaki R, Sano H, et al. Pulmonary hemodynamics and six-minute walk test outcomes in patients with interstitial lung disease. Can Respir J 2016;2016:3837182.

9. Taylor RS, Walker S, Smart NA, et al. Impact of exercise rehabilitation on exercise capacity and quality-of-life in heart failure: individual participant meta-analysis. J Am Coll Cardiol 2019;73(12):1430–43.

10. Farber HW, Miller DP, McGoon MD, et al. Predicting outcomes in pulmonary arterial hypertension based on the 6-minute walk distance. J Heart Lung Transplant 2015;34(3):362–8.

11. Paciocco G, Martinez FJ, Bossone E, et al. Oxygen desaturation on the six-minute walk test and mortality in untreated primary pulmonary hypertension. Eur Respir J 2001;17(4):647–52.

12. Humbert M, Sitbon O, Chaouat A, et al. Survival in patients with idiopathic, familial, and anorexigen-associated pulmonary arterial hypertension in the modern management era. Circulation 2010;122(2):156–63.

13. Benza RL, Miller DP, Gomberg-Maitland M, et al. Predicting survival in pulmonary arterial hypertension: insights from the registry to evaluate early and long-term pulmonary arterial hypertension disease management (REVEAL). Circulation 2010;122(2):164–72.

14. Souza R, Channick RN, Delcroix M, et al. Association between six-minute walk distance and long-term outcomes in patients with pulmonary arterial hypertension: data from the randomized SERAPHIN trial. PLoS One 2018;13(3):e0193226.

15. Mereles D, Ehlken N, Kreuscher S, et al. Exercise and respiratory training improve exercise capacity and quality of life in patients with severe chronic pulmonary hypertension. Circulation 2006;114(14):1482–9.

16. Yock PG, Popp RL. Noninvasive estimation of right ventricular systolic pressure by Doppler ultrasound in patients with tricuspid regurgitation. Circulation 1984;70(4):657–62.

17. Rudski LG, Lai WW, Afilalo J, et al. Guidelines for the echocardiographic assessment of the right heart in adults: a report from the American Society of Echocardiography endorsed by the European Association of Echocardiography, a registered branch of the European Society of Cardiology, and the Canadian Society of Echocardiography. J Am Soc Echocardiogr 2010;23(7):685–713.

18. Humbert M, Kovacs G, Hoeper MM, et al. 2022 ESC/ERS Guidelines for the diagnosis and treatment of pulmonary hypertension. Eur Heart J 2022;43(38):3618–731.

19. D'Alto M, Bossone E, Opotowsky AR, et al. Strengths and weaknesses of echocardiography for the diagnosis of pulmonary hypertension. Int J Cardiol 2018;263:177–83.

20. Vonk NA, et al. The relationship between the right ventricle and its load in pulmonary hypertension. J Am Coll Cardiol 2017;69(2):236–43.

21. Guazzi M, Bandera F, Pelissero G, et al. Tricuspid annular plane systolic excursion and pulmonary arterial systolic pressure relationship in heart failure: an index of right ventricular contractile function and prognosis. Am J Physiol Heart Circ Physiol 2013;305(9):H1373–81.

22. Tello K, Axmann J, Ghofrani HA, et al. Relevance of the TAPSE/PASP ratio in pulmonary arterial hypertension. Int J Cardiol 2018;266:229–35.

23. Tello K, Wan J, Dalmer A, et al. Validation of the tricuspid annular plane systolic excursion/systolic pulmonary artery pressure ratio for the assessment of right ventricular-arterial coupling in severe pulmonary hypertension. Circ Cardiovasc Imaging 2019;12(9):e009047.

24. Herve P, Lau EM, Sitbon O, et al. Criteria for diagnosis of exercise pulmonary hypertension. Eur Respir J 2015;46(3):728–37.

25. Kovacs G, Herve P, Barbera JA, et al. An official European Respiratory Society statement: pulmonary haemodynamics during exercise. Eur Respir J 2017;50(5):1700578.

26. Ho JE, Zern EK, Lau ES, et al. Exercise pulmonary hypertension predicts clinical outcomes in patients with dyspnea on effort. J Am Coll Cardiol 2020;75(1):17–26.

27. Douschan P, Avian A, Foris V, et al. Prognostic value of exercise as compared to resting pulmonary hypertension in patients with normal or mildly elevated pulmonary arterial pressure. Am J Respir Crit Care Med 2022;206(11):1418–23.

28. Rudski LG, et al. Stressing the cardiopulmonary vascular system: the role of echocardiography. J Am Soc Echocardiogr 2018;31(5):527–50.e11.

29. Gargani L, Pugliese NR, De Biase N, et al. Exercise stress echocardiography of the right ventricle and pulmonary circulation. J Am Coll Cardiol 2023;82(21):1973–85.

30. Lancellotti P, Pellikka PA, Budts W, et al. The clinical use of stress echocardiography in non-ischaemic heart disease: recommendations from the European Association of Cardiovascular Imaging and the American Society of Echocardiography. Eur Heart J Cardiovasc Imaging 2016;17(11):1191–229.

31. Douschan P, Tello K, Rieth AJ, et al. Right ventricular-pulmonary arterial coupling and its relationship to exercise haemodynamics in a continuum of patients with pulmonary vascular disease due to chronic thromboembolism. Eur Respir J 2022; 60(3):2200450.

32. Grünig E, Weissmann S, Ehlken N, et al. Stress Doppler echocardiography in relatives of patients with idiopathic and familial pulmonary arterial hypertension: results of a multicenter European analysis of pulmonary artery pressure response to exercise and hypoxia. Circulation 2009;119(13):1747–57.

33. Grünig E, Tiede H, Enyimayew EO, et al. Assessment and prognostic relevance of right ventricular contractile reserve in patients with severe pulmonary hypertension. Circulation 2013;128(18):2005–15.

34. Nagel C, Henn P, Ehlken N, et al. Stress Doppler echocardiography for early detection of systemic sclerosis-associated pulmonary arterial hypertension. Arthritis Res Ther 2015;17(1):165.

35. Douschan P, Kovacs G, Sassmann T, et al. Pulmonary vascular disease and exercise hemodynamics in chronic liver disease. Respir Med 2022;202: 106987.

36. Seeger W, Adir Y, Barberà JA, et al. Pulmonary hypertension in chronic lung diseases. J Am Coll Cardiol 2013;62(25 Suppl):D109–16.

37. Sabbahi A, Severin R, Ozemek C, et al. The role of cardiopulmonary exercise testing and training in patients with pulmonary hypertension: making the case for this assessment and intervention to be considered a standard of care. Expet Rev Respir Med 2020;14(3):317–27.

38. Farina S, Correale M, Bruno N, et al. The role of cardiopulmonary exercise tests in pulmonary arterial hypertension. Eur Respir Rev 2018;27(148):170134.

39. Arena R, Lavie CJ, Milani RV, et al. Cardiopulmonary exercise testing in patients with pulmonary arterial hypertension: an evidence-based review. J Heart Lung Transplant 2010;29(2):159–73.

40. Sun XG, Hansen JE, Oudiz RJ, et al. Exercise pathophysiology in patients with primary pulmonary hypertension. Circulation 2001;104(4):429–35.

41. Weatherald J, Farina S, Bruno N, et al. Cardiopulmonary exercise testing in pulmonary hypertension. Ann Am Thorac Soc 2017;14(Supplement_1):S84–92.

42. Tan X, Yang W, Guo J, et al. Usefulness of decrease in oxygen uptake efficiency to identify gas exchange abnormality in patients with idiopathic pulmonary arterial hypertension. PLoS One 2014;9(6):e98889.

43. Zhao QH, Wang L, Pudasaini B, et al. Cardiopulmonary exercise testing improves diagnostic specificity in patients with echocardiography-suspected pulmonary hypertension. Clin Cardiol 2017;40(2): 95–101.

44. Paolillo S, Farina S, Bussotti M, et al. Exercise testing in the clinical management of patients affected by pulmonary arterial hypertension. Eur J Prev Cardiol 2012;19(5):960–71.

45. Mollet NR, Cademartiri F, de Feyter PJ. Non-invasive multislice CT coronary imaging. Heart 2005;91(3): 401–7.

46. Cademartiri F, Runza G, Belgrano M, et al. Introduction to coronary imaging with 64-slice computed tomography. Radiol Med 2005;110(1–2):16–41.

47. Cademartiri F, Luccichenti G, Marano R, et al. Spiral CT-angiography with one, four, and sixteen slice scanners. Technical note. Radiol Med 2003;106(4): 269–83.

48. Cademartiri F, Luccichenti G, Marano R, et al. Non-invasive angiography of the coronary arteries with multislice computed tomography: state of the art and future prospects. Radiol Med 2003;106(4): 284–96.

49. Cademartiri F, Casolo G, Clemente A, et al. Coronary CT angiography: a guide to examination, interpretation, and clinical indications. Expert Rev Cardiovasc Ther 2021;19(5):413–25.

50. Cademartiri F, Maurovich-Horvat P. Current role of coronary calcium in younger population and future prospects with photon counting technology. Eur Heart J Cardiovasc Imaging 2022;24(1):25–6.

51. Meloni A, Cademartiri F, Positano V, et al. Cardiovascular applications of photon-counting CT technology: a revolutionary new diagnostic step. J Cardiovasc Dev Dis 2023;10(9):363.

52. Meloni A, Frijia F, Panetta D, et al. Photon-Counting computed tomography (PCCT): technical background and cardio-vascular applications. Diagnostics (Basel) 2023;13(4):645.

53. Cademartiri F, Meloni A, Pistoia L, et al. Dual-source photon-counting computed tomography-Part I: clinical overview of cardiac CT and coronary CT angiography applications. J Clin Med 2023;12(11):3627.

54. Cademartiri F, Meloni A, Pistoia L, et al. Dual source photon-counting computed tomography-Part II: clinical overview of neurovascular applications. J Clin Med 2023;12(11):3626.

55. Meloni A, Cademartiri F, Pistoia L, et al. Dual-source photon-counting computed tomography-Part III: clinical overview of vascular applications beyond cardiac and neuro imaging. J Clin Med 2023; 12(11):3798.

56. Zanon C, Cademartiri F, Toniolo A, et al. Advantages of photon-counting detector CT in aortic imaging. Tomography 2023;10(1):1–13.

57. Schoepf UJ, Helmberger T, Holzknecht N, et al. Segmental and subsegmental pulmonary arteries: evaluation with electron-beam versus spiral CT. Radiology 2000;214(2):433–9.

58. Schoepf UJ, Holzknecht N, Helmberger TK, et al. Subsegmental pulmonary emboli: improved detection with thin-collimation multi-detector row spiral CT. Radiology 2002;222(2):483–90.

59. Herzog P, Wildberger JE, Niethammer M, et al. CT perfusion imaging of the lung in pulmonary embolism. Acad Radiol 2003;10(10):1132–46.

60. Zhou Y, Shi H, Wang Y, et al. Assessment of correlation between CT angiographic clot load score, pulmonary perfusion defect score and global right ventricular function with dual-source CT for acute pulmonary embolism. Br J Radiol 2012;85(1015): 972–9.

61. Li K, Li Y, Qi Z, et al. Quantitative lung perfusion blood volume using dual energy CT-based effective atomic number (Z_{eff}) imaging. Med Phys 2021; 48(11):6658–72.

62. Maffei E, Messalli G, Martini C, et al. Left and right ventricle assessment with Cardiac CT: validation study vs. Cardiac MR. Eur Radiol 2012;22(5): 1041–9.

63. Takx RA, Moscariello A, Schoepf UJ, et al. Quantification of left and right ventricular function and myocardial mass: comparison of low-radiation dose 2nd generation dual-source CT and cardiac MRI. Eur J Radiol 2012;81(4):e598–604.

64. Swift AJ, Dwivedi K, Johns C, et al. Diagnostic accuracy of CT pulmonary angiography in suspected pulmonary hypertension. Eur Radiol 2020;30(9): 4918–29.

65. Nootens M, Wolfkiel CJ, Chomka EV, et al. Understanding right and left ventricular systolic function and interactions at rest and with exercise in primary pulmonary hypertension. Am J Cardiol 1995;75(5): 374–7.

66. Hamirani YS, Kramer CM. Advances in stress cardiac MRI and computed tomography. Future Cardiol 2013;9(5):681–95.

67. Grothues F, Moon JC, Bellenger NG, et al. Interstudy reproducibility of right ventricular volumes, function, and mass with cardiovascular magnetic resonance. Am Heart J 2004;147(2):218–23.

68. Lahm T, Douglas IS, Archer SL, et al. Assessment of right ventricular function in the research setting: knowledge gaps and pathways forward. An official American thoracic society research statement. Am J Respir Crit Care Med 2018;198(4):e15–43.

69. Hudsmith LE, Petersen SE, Francis JM, et al. Normal human left and right ventricular and left atrial dimensions using steady state free precession magnetic resonance imaging. J Cardiovasc Magn Reson 2005;7(5):775–82.

70. Rehwald WG, Fieno DS, Chen EL, et al. Myocardial magnetic resonance imaging contrast agent concentrations after reversible and irreversible ischemic injury. Circulation 2002;105(2):224–9.

71. McLaughlin VV, Presberg KW, Doyle RL, et al. Prognosis of pulmonary arterial hypertension: ACCP evidence-based clinical practice guidelines. Chest 2004;126(1 Suppl):78S–92S.

72. Alabed S, Shahin Y, Garg P, et al. Cardiac-MRI predicts clinical worsening and mortality in pulmonary arterial hypertension: a systematic review and meta-analysis. JACC Cardiovasc Imaging 2021; 14(5):931–42.

73. Goh ZM, Balasubramanian N, Alabed S, et al. Right ventricular remodelling in pulmonary arterial hypertension predicts treatment response. Heart 2022; 108(17):1392–400.

74. de Siqueira ME, Pozo E, Fernandes VR, et al. Characterization and clinical significance of right ventricular mechanics in pulmonary hypertension evaluated with cardiovascular magnetic resonance feature tracking. J Cardiovasc Magn Reson 2016; 18(1):39.

75. Tello K, Dalmer A, Vanderpool R, et al. Cardiac magnetic resonance imaging-based right ventricular strain analysis for assessment of coupling and diastolic function in pulmonary hypertension. JACC Cardiovasc Imaging 2019;12(11 Pt 1):2155–64.

76. Swift AJ, Rajaram S, Capener D, et al. LGE patterns in pulmonary hypertension do not impact overall mortality. JACC Cardiovasc Imaging 2014;7(12): 1209–17.

77. Trankle CR, Canada JM, Jordan JH, et al. Exercise cardiovascular magnetic resonance: a review. J Magn Reson Imaging 2022;55(3):720–54.

The Invasive Cardiopulmonary Exercise Test: A Practical Guide

Scott H. Visovatti, MD[a],*, Bradley A. Maron, MD[b,c]

KEYWORDS

- Exercise intolerance • Cardiopulmonary exercise test • Hemodynamics
- Right heart catheterization • CPET • iCPET

KEY POINTS

- The invasive cardiopulmonary exercise test (iCPET) provides a comprehensive assessment of an individual's hemodynamic, ventilatory, and gas exchange responses to exercise. The data gathered during a high-quality iCPET are helpful in both diagnosing and deeply phenotyping the conditions contributing to exercise intolerance.
- Though the iCPET is a complex test, a well-coordinated, multidisciplinary team–based approach to performing the test produces accurate, clinically useful results. It is essential that each iCPET is performed using a thoughtful, detailed protocol that leverages the local expertise of the team performing the iCPET test.
- Given that a standardized approach to performing an iCPET does not exist, each program must carefully consider essential topics including safety precautions, zero referencing of the pulmonary arterial catheter, body position during exercise, interpretation of waveforms during exercise, and the means of measuring cardiac output when creating a protocol.

INTRODUCTION

The invasive cardiopulmonary exercise test (iCPET) provides a comprehensive assessment of ventilatory, cardiac, pulmonary vascular, metabolic, or multifactorial limitations to exercise, and many consider it to be the "gold standard" test for the evaluation of dyspnea of unknown origin.[1] The noninvasive cardiopulmonary exercise test (CPET) has long been used to evaluate the contribution of conditions such as heart failure, chronic obstructive pulmonary disease, interstitial lung disease, pulmonary vascular disease, cystic fibrosis, and exercise-induced bronchospasm to an individual's exercise intolerance.[2] In addition, CPET has played an important role in the selection of patients for cardiac and lung transplantation,

the development of plans for cardiac and pulmonary rehabilitation programs, and the assessment of response to therapy in patients with respiratory or cardiovascular diseases.[2] Incorporating hemodynamic assessment over the course of an exercise study enables iCPET results to assist clinicians identify conditions that are challenging or impossible to diagnose at rest, including exercise postcapillary pulmonary hypertension,[3,4] exercise precapillary pulmonary hypertension,[3,4] chronic thromboembolic pulmonary hypertension (CTEPH),[5] and preload limitation to exercise[3,4] (**Fig. 1**). In most instances, the iCPET includes peripheral arterial blood gas (ABG) collection, which allows the assessment of O_2 flux across the skeletal muscle among other pathophysiologic processes. More recently, centers with iCPET

[a] Division of Cardiovascular Medicine, Department of Internal Medicine, The Ohio State University School of Medicine, DHLRI Room 255, 473 West 12th Avenue, Columbus, OH 43210, USA; [b] Department of Medicine, University of Maryland School of Medicine, 6116 Executive Boulevard, North Bethesda, MD 20852, USA; [c] The University of Maryland-Institute for Health Computing, Baltimore, MD, USA
* Corresponding author.
E-mail address: Scott.Visovatti@osumc.edu

Heart Failure Clin 21 (2025) 79–91
https://doi.org/10.1016/j.hfc.2024.08.002
1551-7136/25/© 2024 Elsevier Inc. All rights reserved, including those for text and data mining, AI training, and similar technologies.

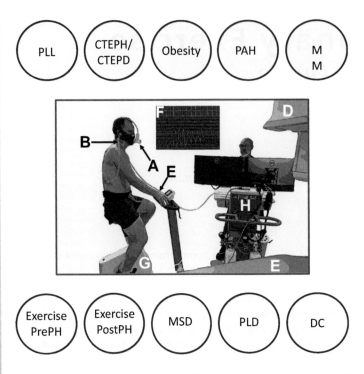

Fig. 1. Limitations to exercise and the invasive cardiopulmonary exercise test. The iCPET involves a PA catheter, RA catheter, and metabolic cart to assess the cardiovascular, respiratory, and metabolic responses to exercise. The findings are helpful in identifying a variety of limitations to exercise, including pulmonary arterial hypertension (PAH), exercise precapillary and postcapillary pulmonary hypertension, chronic thromboembolic pulmonary hypertension, chronic thromboembolic pulmonary disease, preload limitation to exercise, pulmonary mechanical limitation to exercise, mitochondrial myopathy, and deconditioning. Essential equipment includes a mask and a mouthpiece (A), PA catheter (B) placed in a cath lab using a fluoroscope (C) while the patient is supine on a table (D), RA line (E), hemodynamic recording system (F), ergometer (G), and metabolic cart (H). DC, deconditioning; Exercise PostPH, exercise postcapillary pulmonary hypertension; Exercise PrePH, exercise precapillary pulmonary hypertension; iCPET, invasive cardiopulmonary exercise test; LD, parenchymal lung disease; MSD, muscular-skeletal disease; MM, mitochondrial myopathy; PLL, preload limitation; PHA, pulmonary arterial hypertension.

expertise are leveraging the test to phenotype conditions, including pulmonary arterial hypertension,[6] myalgic encephalomyelitis/chronic fatigue syndrome,[7] and exercise limitations in patients following coronavirus disease infection.[8–11] In the research domain, investigators have used iCPET variables to develop point-of-care risk stratification tools for patients with exercise intolerance[12] and designed clinical trials using iCPET parameters as the primary endpoints.[13]

Given the utility of the test, there is great interest in establishing iCPET programs. However, the complexity of performing and interpreting the study can appear daunting. While previous publications have provided excellent, high-level overviews of how to perform the iCPET,[3,4,6,14] our aim in this article is to provide an in-depth description of how to set up and perform the test. Our hope is that this information helps to demystify the iCPET and provide cardiologists, pulmonologists, and exercise physiologists with information necessary for the performance of high-quality, interpretable studies.

THE INVASIVE CARDIOPULMONARY EXERCISE TEST PROTOCOL

As shown in **Fig. 2**, a high-quality iCPET requires a regimented protocol involving a gradually increasing work rate because of the increasing pedal resistance during cycle ergometry. A ramp protocol is generally used, and the optimal increase in work rate can either be calculated[15] or estimated. For example, the pulmonary vascular disease phenomics (PVDOMICS) protocol assigns patients to 1 of the 3 continuous ramp protocols, depending upon their functional status: a 10-W increase per two-minute interval is used if the patient becomes dyspneic or fatigued when walking from room to room at home; a 15-W increase per two-minute interval is employed if the patient can walk from room to room at home without difficulty but experiences dyspnea or fatigue when climbing a single flight of stairs; a 20-W increase per two-minute interval is used if the patient can climb one flight of stairs without difficulty.[6] Patients pedal at a rate of 60 revolutions per minute. Continuous assessment of gas exchange parameters occurs over the course of the study, and collection of additional data (eg, hemodynamics, blood gas, respiratory exchange ratio, symptom assessment) occurs at prespecified time points. The process repeats until the subject reaches adequate exercise effort, cannot continue because of symptoms, or experiences an indication for early termination of exercise (**Box 1**). A determination of adequate exercise effort is generally made in part by monitoring the ratio of CO_2 output to O_2 uptake (VCO_2/VO_2) over the course of exercise. This respiratory exchange ratio (RER) rises quickly after a subject crosses the anaerobic threshold because of a rapid rise in CO_2; many

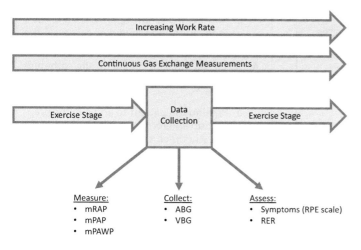

Fig. 2. iCPET study sequence. The iCPET is performed using an ergometer with gradually increasing resistance. Each stage is defined by a predetermined amount of time (generally 2 minutes). After each stage, invasive hemodynamics are measured, blood gasses (arterial and mixed venous) are collected, and symptoms are assessed using the RPE scale. Gas exchange parameters are collected continuously over the course of the study. AGB, arterial blood gas; mPAP, mean pulmonary arterial pressure; mPAWP, mean pulmonary artery wedge pressure; mRAP, mean right atrial pressure; RER, respiratory exchange ratio; RPE, Rating of Preserved Exertion; VBG, venous blood gas (a mixed venous sample from the pulmonary artery).

protocols use an RER greater than 1.16 (unless the patient is hyperventilating), combined with the VCO_2/VO_2 slope, to determine when a patient has reached an adequate exercise effort.[15]

No standard iCPET protocol exists, and each center performs the test with some variability.

Nascent iCPET programs often develop protocols after team members observe studies at established centers and then take their own needs and expertise into account. A detailed example of an iCPET protocol is provided in **Box 2**. It is important to note that protocols are often modified over time as centers develop expertise, leverage center-specific resources, and address local clinical needs. Another valuable resource that shows the components of an actual iCPET at an established center is an online video supplement by Berry and colleagues[3]

INVASIVE CARDIOPULMONARY EXERCISE TEST INTERPRETATION

A high-quality iCPET produces a great deal of data, and a comprehensive evaluation of the data requires multidisciplinary expertise, considerable time, and an understanding of how the hemodynamic and gas exchange patterns produced through testing implicate specific disease states in a patient's exercise intolerance. It is recommended that a multidisciplinary team–based approach to iCPET analysis be used.[16] Ideally, the iCPET team should bring together individuals with considerable domain expertise in CPET and exercise right heart catheterizations (RHCs). This type of multidisciplinary team is also uniquely positioned to generate the kind of questions and hypotheses that lead to research initiatives within an iCPET program. As the program grows, it is likely that individual providers will gain the experience necessary to fully analyze iCPET data without involvement from a multidisciplinary team.

Excellent overviews of iCPET interpretation have been published,[3,4,14] and practical approaches to gas exchange interpretation have been published[17,18] or are available online.[5]

Box 2
Invasive cardiopulmonary exercise test (iCPET) protocol

1. Upon receiving an order for an iCPET,

   a. The iCPET team reviews the patient's chart to determine

      i. If the study is capable of answering the clinical question posed; this may require a conversation with the referring provider,

      ii. If there are absolute or relative contraindications to exercise testing (see **Table 1**),

      iii. If pertinent studies have been performed within the previous 6 months, including

         1. A stress test,

         2. An echocardiogram,

         3. A pulmonary function test (ideally, a full study),

         4. A left heart catheterization with coronary angiogram,

         5. A right heart catheterization (at rest)

2. The iCPET team contacts the patient to

   a. Provide an overview of the study,

   b. Determine whether the patient is on supplemental oxygen (an iCPET performed on supplemental oxygen requires the use of a Douglas bag),

   c. Determine if any of the following is suspected:

      i. Inability to exercise using the ergometer

      ii. Inability to exercise to an extent that will allow the patient to cross the anaerobic threshold

      iii. Inability to form a tight seal with the mouthpiece

   d. Ask the patient to bring the following items on the day of the study:

      i. Track pants/sweat pants or similar loose fitting pants to wear under a hospital gown

      ii. Sports bra (for women)

      iii. Gym/workout shoes

3. Following the patient call, the iCPET team will either

   a. Contact the exercise physiology team and catheterization lab schedulers to coordinate a study date.

   b. Contact the referring provider and catheterization lab schedulers to cancel the study request.

4. Seven days before the iCPET, the catheterization lab preparation team will call the patient to

   a. Remind the patient to arrive in the preparation and recovery area 2 hours before the scheduled study time.

   b. Remind the patient to continue all medications, with the exception of anticoagulants and diuretics. The iCPET team may ask that additional medications be held on a case-by-case basis.

   c. Ask that they have a driver on the day of the iCPET.

   d. Answer any last-minute questions.

   e. Remind the patient that a light breakfast is permitted.

5. Day of study: procedure preparation (before the patient arrives in the catheterization lab)

   a. Prepare radial artery (ABG) and pulmonary artery (VBG) blood gas sample syringes

      i. Preprint stickers for syringes

         1. Printed on each sticker is

            a. The patient's name and medical record number

            b. The stage at which the sample will be drawn. For example, the ABG drawn during the first stage is designated "A1", while the VBG drawn during the first stage is designated "V1"

         2. Generally, 7 ABG and 7 VBG stickers are prepared; the number can be adjusted based upon the expected duration of exercise

      ii. The anticipated number of ABG and VBG syringes are removed from their wrappers, placed on a small table, and covered with a sterile drape

   b. Metabolic cart preparation

      i. The vacuum pump is started at least 30 minutes before the patient enters the room

      ii. The metabolic cart is calibrated, per manufacturer's recommendations

      iii. *Note*: depending upon the catheterization lab availability before the iCPET, the above 2 steps may need to be performed in a staging area. The prepared metabolic cart can then be brought into the catheterization lab immediately before the study

c. Procedure table preparation. The following materials are placed on the table:

  i. Sterile towels

  ii. Sharp container

  iii. Sterile syringes (multiple 10 cc and 20 cc)

  iv. 4x4 gauze

  v. Liquid waste cup

  vi. Patient drape

  vii. Band-Aid

  viii. Sterile gloves

  ix. Sterile ultrasound probe cover

  x. 2% buffered lidocaine in a 10 cc syringe with 25G needle

  xi. Cook Micropuncture Access Set (21Gx7 cm needle, 4-Frx10 cm outer catheter, 0.018" Dx40 cm guide wire). Part number G48003

  xii. Retractable scalpel

  xiii. 8-Fr sheath with access wire

  xiv. Swan-Ganz Fr thermodilution pulmonary arterial catheter

  xv. Pulmonary arterial catheter protective sleeve (Teleflex Arrow TwistLock Catheter Contamination Shield-Gard, 8.5 Fr x 80 cm locks on to 8-Fr sheath

  xvi. Pulmonary arterial catheter securement dressing (3M Tegaderm IV Advanced Securement Dressing, product number 1688)

  xvii. VBG collection setup (used to collect samples from distal port of the pulmonary arterial catheter)

    1. "Double gang" setup as described in **Fig. 1**C of "How to Start an Invasive Cardiopulmonary Exercise Testing Program: A Comprehensive and Practical Guide" by Michael G. Risbano in this issue of Heart Failure Clinics

    a. Two 3-way stop cocks

    b. Two Luer Lock adapters

    c. 10-cc Luer Lock syringe

    d. 0.9% sterile normal saline bag (500 cc)

    e. Tubing for connecting saline bag to double gang setup

  xviii. ABG collection setup (used to collect samples from the radial arterial catheter)

    1. Radial artery placement kit (such as the Arrow 20 Gauge x 4.45 cm kit (SKU NA-04020)

    2. Tegaderm for securing arterial catheter

    3. VAMP adult closed blood sampling system (Edwards 48VMP120)

    4. VAMP system needless canula (Edwards VMP 400)

    5. 0.9% sterile normal saline (500 cc)

    6. A TR Band for postprocedural hemostasis after arterial catheter is removed

d. ABG/VBG access stand

  i. ABG/VBG syringes x 14 covered with drape (as described in 5a)

e. Nonsterile items

  i. Ultrasound machine and probe

  ii. Skin marker

  iii. IV pole on wheels

  iv. Laser level attached to a transducer holder capable of holding 3 transducers for radial arterial, right atrial (RA), and pulmonary arterial (PA) pressure measurements (see **Fig. 3**A, B)

6. Day of study: patient in the preparation area

  a. A history and physical is performed

  b. A sedation assessment is performed (local anesthetic is used for the right internal jugular sheath and radial arterial line catheter placements; conscious sedation not permitted).

  c. An overview of the iCPET is provided.

  d. An Allen test is performed to make sure it is safe to place a radial artery catheter in the catheterization lab.

  e. Informed consent is obtained.

7. Day of study: study preparation with patient in the procedure room

  a. The patient is seated in a recliner chair behind the ergometer.

  b. Standard catheterization lab "time out" policies regarding introductions, patient identification, pertinent laboratory values, study overview, and questions or concerns are followed.

c. Electrocardiogram electrodes are placed. In some systems, 2 sets of electrodes are needed (one for the catheterization lab hemodynamic recording system and one for the metabolic cart).

d. The patient is seated on the ergometer, and seat height is adjusted

   i. The knee should be slightly bent (20° angle) at the bottom of a pedal stroke.

e. Transducer leveling preparation is performed (see **Fig. 3**)

   i. A laser level attached to an adjustable transducer holder is mounted on an IV pole.

   ii. While seated on the ergometer, a skin marker is used to mark a horizontal line 3 finger widths below the axilla. This mark is transferred to the patient's back using the laser level/transducer holder device mounted to a rolling IV pole.

   iii. The mid-axillary line, perpendicular to the first line, is also marked.

   iv. The laser level/transducer holder device is adjusted to the level of the horizontal line while the patient is seated on the ergometer and then while seated in a recliner chair behind the ergometer. The height of these 2 positions is marked on the IV pole using a tape, allowing for rapid adjustments and height adjustments of the transducers later in the case.

f. While seated in the recliner chair, the maximum voluntary ventilation is measured.

g. The patient is escorted to the catheterization lab table and situated in a supine position.

h. The height of the catheterization lab table is adjusted to a height that allows for placement of the radial arterial and pulmonary arterial catheters.

   i. *Note*: It is important that no adjustments to the height of the table be made after this point, as doing so will alter the relationship between the patient and the pressure transducers mounted to the IV pole (and thus alter pressure measurements).

j. The laser level/transducer holder device is adjusted to align with the previously marked mid-axillary line.

k. The EKG lead cables of the catheterization lab hemodynamic recording system are attached to the electrodes.

8. Day of study: radial arterial line placement

   a. A radial arm is used to place the left wrist in the optimal position for radial arterial access.

   b. Arterial line tubing and VAMP system are prepped.

   c. Arterial catheter is placed with ultrasound guidance.

   d. Tubing and VAMP system are connected to the arterial catheter

   e. The arterial catheter is secured using small Tegaderms both above and below the arterial line (the catheter is not sutured into place).

   f. The system is connected to a transducer on the IV pole.

9. Day of study: resting hemodynamic measurements

   a. The patient is prepped and draped in sterile usual fashion for right internal jugular vein access.

   b. Access is obtained using the Micropuncture kit and ultrasound guidance.

   c. An 8-Fr sheath is placed. *Note*: the sheath hub is not sutured to the patient.

   d. A pulmonary arterial catheter protective sleeve is placed over a flushed and prepped 7-Fr Swan-Ganz thermodilution pulmonary arterial catheter, and the catheter is introduced through the sheath.

   e. The following are measured while the patient is supine and at rest:

      i. Hemodynamics:

         1. Right atrial pressures (RAP)

         2. Right ventricular pressures (RVP)

         3. Pulmonary arterial pressures (PAP)

         4. Pulmonary arterial wedge pressures (PAWP)

      ii. Cardiac output and index using:

         1. The thermodilution method

         2. The Direct Fick method (using mixed venous and radial arterial oxygen saturations)

      iii. Oxygen saturations: superior vena cava, pulmonary arterial, and radial arterial saturation. A full shunt run may be performed at this time, if appropriate.

f. Once the resting study is completed, final positioning of the pulmonary arterial catheter is performed so that the PAWP is easily obtained. This must take into account the tendency of the catheter to dive deeper into the pulmonary artery during exercise.

g. A sterile pulmonary arterial catheter securement dressing is applied.

h. The pulmonary arterial catheter protective sleeve is locked to the sheath hub.

i. The RA lumen from the pulmonary catheter is flushed and then connected to the RA transducer on the laser level/transducer holder assembly.

j. The PA lumen from the pulmonary catheter is flushed and then connected to the double gang system (described in 5.C.xvii), which is connected in series to the PA transducer on the laser level/transducer holder assembly.

k. Any additional lumens from the pulmonary catheter are flushed and capped.

l. Care is taken to make sure the balloon on the pulmonary arterial catheter is deflated, the inflation port is in the locked position, and the inflation syringe is tightly connected to the port.

10. Day of study: preexercise setup and measurements

a. The patient is escorted from the catheterization table to the recliner chair behind the ergometer. *Note*: Care must be taken to make sure there will be no tension in any of the lines leading to transducers when the patient moves from the catheterization table to the recliner.

b. The EKG lead cables for the metabolic cart are connected to the appropriate electrodes.

c. The laser level/transducer holder assembly is lowered to the tape line on the IV pole corresponding to the chair position, as described in 7.f.iv and shown in **Fig. 3**E.

d. The exercise physiology team provides instructions to the patient including

i. The importance of not talking while the mouthpiece is in place.

ii. The importance of using the Rate of Perceived Exertion Scale to relay information about symptoms during the test.

iii. The importance of not abruptly stopping exercise and the need for a cool down period following the end of exercise.

e. The mouthpiece is fitted to the patient, and preexercise/resting gas exchange values are obtained.

f. The following resting hemodynamic values are obtained while seated in the chair:

i. RAP

ii. PAP

iii. PAWP

g. Seated resting PA and RA saturations are drawn.

h. Last-minute instructions are given, and any questions are answered

i. The patient is escorted to the ergometer, optimal seat height is confirmed, and the patient's feet are slipped under the pedal straps.

j. The exercise physiology team reviews instructions regarding the exercise study and reminds the patient that cooling down is essential to help prevent syncope.

k. The laser level/transducer assembly is adjusted to the previously identified level.

11. Day of study: exercise study

a. The phases of the exercise study are the following:

i. Resting in chair. After 2 minutes, hemodynamics are measured and blood gasses drawn.

ii. Resting on ergometer. After 2 minutes, hemodynamics are measured and blood gasses drawn.

iii. Warm up. This uses the "freewheel" setting, during which the ergometer drives the pedals for 2 minutes. After 2 minutes, hemodynamics are measured and blood gasses drawn.

iv. Exercise stages (2 minutes each). After 2 minutes, hemodynamics are measured and blood gasses drawn.

v. Cooldown. Three-minute cooldown on ergometer (legs keep moving, no hemodynamics are measured or blood gasses drawn)

vi. Recovery. The patient is moved to the chair immediately after cooldown, and the final hemodynamic measurements and blood gas draws are performed. *Note*: Recovery should not take place on the ergometer as syncope can occur immediately after the legs stop moving.

b. The sequence of events for each exercise stage is the following:

  i. The exercise physiologist calls out and records the time

    1. The following hemodynamics are recorded (2 respiratory cycles):

      a. RAP

      b. PAP

      c. PAWP (requires inflation of PA catheter balloon). *Note*: the PA catheter may dive deeper into PA during exercise than it does at rest. Monitor the PA waveform throughout exercise to make sure it does not self-wedge during exercise. If self-wedging is noted, the PA catheter should be pulled back to prevent this. The team should also monitor the PAWP during balloon inflation to make sure over-wedging is not occurring.

  ii. Waste is drawn from the radial arterial line and PA catheter lumen (this is most performed using the double gang set-up for the PA catheter and VAMP system for the RA catheter)

  iii. The following blood gasses are drawn at exactly the same time

    1. A VBG sample from the PA catheter

    2. An ABG sample from the RA catheter

    3. *Note*: Once drawn, the exercise physiologist records the exact time so that the blood gas results can be used to calculate a direct Fick cardiac output using the Vo_2 at the specific time of the blood draws.

  iv. The PA catheter and RA catheters are flushed

c. ABG and VBG sample processing

  i. The samples are run to the central lab in batches of 4 samples. *Note*: Specific institutional recommendations should be followed when considering whether blood gas samples should be placed on ice.

  ii. Each sample is analyzed for the following:

    1. pH

    2. $Paco_2$

    3. Pao_2

    4. SaO_2

    5. HCO_3

    6. Lactate

    7. Base excess

    8. Plasma lactate

    9. Hemoglobin

    10. Hematocrit

12. Day of study: posttest

a. Following the final measurements, the following are removed from the patient:

  i. PA catheter

  ii. Right internal jugular sheath (some catheterization lab policies require that this be performed while the patient is supine and exhaling)

  iii. Radial artery catheter

    1. Apply a TR Band compression device

    2. Monitor the patient in the procedural recovery area to assure that hemostasis is achieved and arterial blood flow to the hand remains normal as the TR Band is deflated

Modified from the University of Pittsburgh Advanced Cardiopulmonary Exercise Testing Program.

Comprehensive resources have been published by Sietsema *and colleagues*[15] in the American Thoracic Society/American College of Chest Physicians[2] and the European Respiratory Society.[19] The definition of exercise precapillary pulmonary and exercise postcapillary pulmonary hypertension have varied in recent years; the recent 2022 European Society of Cardiology (ESC)/European Respiratory Society guidelines define the former as a mean pulmonary arterial pressure/cardiac output slope greater than 3 mm Hg/L/min between rest and exercise and the latter as a pulmonary arterial wedge pressure (PAWP)/cardiac output slope greater than 2 mm Hg/L/min.[20]

CONSIDERATIONS
Safety

The iCPET is an invasive study that applies significant stress to individuals who are already experiencing some degree of exercise intolerance. In many cases, the combination of a disease process and deconditioning resulting from that process may make the iCPET the most intense physical activity in which a patient has engaged in quite some time. In fact, complete and accurate evaluation of metabolic gas exchange parameters is generally possible only after a subject has achieved a maximal effort and crossed the anaerobic threshold (as evidenced by a respiratory exchange ratio greater than 1.1).[15] Thus, it is important to make sure that the risk/benefit ratio is in favor of performing maximal exercise testing. This involves assuring that a potential iCPET candidate has undergone a thorough evaluation using appropriate tests at rest, that the iCPET is capable of answering the clinical questions, and that the list of absolute and relative contraindications is reviewed (**Table 1**). In addition, should the decision be made to perform an iCPET, all team members must monitor the patient for indications for exercise termination throughout testing (see **Box 1**).

Though there are no large-scale assessments of the additive risk of performing a RHC during cardiopulmonary exercise testing, expert opinion is that the assessment of exercise hemodynamics poses minimal additional risk compared with a resting RHC.[19] Despite this reassurance, there are several aspects of an iCPET that require close attention. First, vigorous exercise can cause the pulmonary artery (PA) catheter to migrate more distally into the pulmonary vasculature, placing the patient at an increased risk for PA rupture when the balloon is inflated for PAWP measurements. To minimize the risk of rupture, the proceduralist should inflate the balloon slowly using the designated (volume limited) custom syringe and only to the extent necessary to change the PA waveform to a PAWP waveform. In addition, it should not be assumed that the volume of air needed to inflate and wedge the balloon at rest is the same volume required during exercise. Second, placement of a radial arterial catheter (not used at all centers) can result in complications

---

Table 1
Relative and absolute contraindications to iCPET

Absolute	Relative
Acute myocardial infarction (3–5 d)	Left main coronary stenosis or its equivalent
Unstable angina	Moderate stenotic valvular heart disease
Uncontrolled arrhythmias causing symptoms or hemodynamic compromise	Severe untreated arterial hypertension at rest (>200 mm Hg systolic; >120 mmHg diastolic)
Active endocarditis	Tachyarrhythmias or bradyarrhythmias
Acute myocarditis or pericarditis	High-degree AV block
Symptomatic severe aortic stenosis	Hypertrophic cardiomyopathy or other forms of outflow tract obstruction
Decompensated heart failure	Significant pulmonary hypertension
Acute pulmonary embolism or pulmonary infarction	Advanced or complicated pregnancy
Thrombosis of the lower extremities	Electrolyte abnormalities
Suspected dissecting aneurysm	Orthopedic impairment that compromises exercise performance
Uncontrolled asthma	
Pulmonary edema	
Room air desaturation ≤ 85% (unless supplemental oxygen to be administered during exercise)	
Respiratory failure	
Acute noncardiopulmonary disorder that may affect exercise performance or be aggravated by exercise (ie, infection, renal failure, thyrotoxicosis)	
Mental impairment leading to inability to cooperate	

including artery occlusion, perforation, dissection, spasm, hematoma (possibly resulting in compartment syndrome), nerve damage, infection, pseudoaneurysm, and arteriovenous fistula.[21] Use of ultrasound guidance, avoidance of repeated punctures and the use of a TR Band or a similar compression device for hemostasis can help minimize the risk of complications. Third, patients undergoing iCPET are at risk for postexercise syncope because of issues including an exaggerated form of the normal postexercise hypotension response, the Bezold-Jarisch reflex, a vasovagal reaction, or a preload limitation to exercise. Avoiding an abrupt cessation of exercise and not allowing the patient to remain on an upright ergometer following an iCPET can help prevent, or mitigate the repercussions of, postexercise syncope. Many centers require the presence of a reclining chair near the ergometer; this provides a safe "landing spot" for a syncopal or presyncopal patient who needs to be placed in a recumbent position. At our own center, we perform preexercise and immediate postexercise hemodynamic and gas exchange measurements while the patient is sitting in the recliner, which avoids having to perform the postexercise assessment when the patent is sitting upright on the ergometer (and vulnerable to postexercise syncope). As described below and shown in **Fig. 2**, accurate hemodynamic assessments over the course of an iCPET that involves changes in body position (supine, upright on the ergometer, upright in a chair) require a system for meticulous adjustments of transducer height to maintain the zero-reference level.

Zero-Reference Level

The optimal zero-reference level for the PA catheter, during both rest and exercise studies, is the left atrium.[19] For a standard supine resting RHC, it is relatively easy to identify and maintain the zero-reference level (the midthoracic level at the point where the fourth rib inserts into the sternum[19]). However, maintaining the zero-reference level over the course of an iCPET study is much more challenging as many protocols require that the patient moves from a supine position to at least one upright position. To assure that positional changes do not introduce inaccuracy into the hemodynamic measurements, most iCPET programs have developed exacting approaches maintaining the zero-reference level. One such approach is shown in **Fig. 3** and described in **Box 2**.

Essential Hemodynamic Measurements

Expert consensus recommends the measurement of mean pulmonary arterial pressure (mPAP),

PAWP, and cardiac output (CO) at each stage of exercise, as well as the calculation of total pulmonary resistance (mPAP/CO), pulmonary vascular resistance (mPAP-PAWP/CO), and mPAP/CO slope.[19] iCPET teams should also consider measuring (1) pulmonary arterial compliance, which assesses the pressure/volume relationship in the pulmonary vasculature, and is defined as the stroke volume divided by pulmonary arterial pulse pressure (systolic pulmonary arterial pressure – diastolic pulmonary arterial pressure); (2) right ventricular stroke work index, which reflects right ventricular function, and is defined as the mPAP minus the right atrial pressure multiplied by the stroke volume divided by the body surface area.[22] Calculation of the PAWP/CO slope over the course of the study can be helpful in helping to diagnose diastolic dysfunction.

Upright Versus Supine Ergometer

iCPET studies are performed using either an upright or a supine ergometer; each of these options has advantages and disadvantages. A supine iCPET allows for the use of fluoroscopy during the test, if needed (such as when there is concern that the PA catheter is diving too deep with exercise and over-wedging). In addition, the patient does not need to change position from supine (for the resting RHC) to upright (for the exercise portion of the study); this obviates the need for meticulous adjustment of the transducers to assure that the zero-reference level is maintained. However, a supine study requires raising of the legs above the level of the heart, reducing the perfusion pressure and muscle oxygen delivery-to-uptake ratio.[23] These changes may result in a lower work rate achieved by the time the patient experiences symptom-limited cessation of the test. Finally, the diagnosis of pulmonary hypertension, a condition that is often considered in patients with exertional dyspnea, is based upon hemodynamic values measure in the supine position at rest.[20]

The decision to perform an iCPET in an upright position is often based upon the desire to evaluate responses to exercise in the position that approximates an individual's most common daily posture. As discussed by Sarma in his article in this volume, changes in chest wall compliance are more significant in the supine position compared with the upright position, and can increase both pleural pressure and PCWP. Such effects are more pronounced in patients with obesity or respiratory diseases, and thus performing an iCPET in the upright position may provide more accurate PAWP measurements in these patient populations. Studies

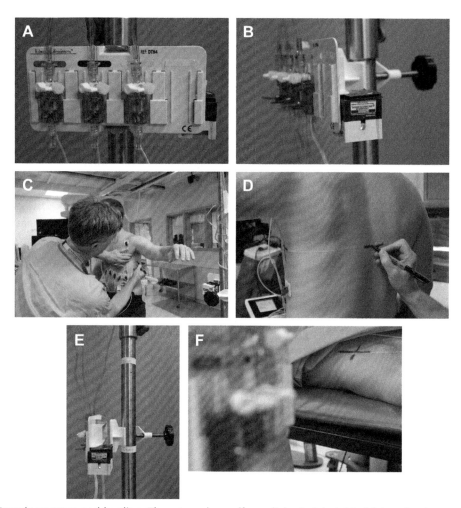

Fig. 3. Transducer setup and leveling. Three transducers (for radial arterial, right atrial, and pulmonary arterial pressure measurements) are placed in a standard holder (*A*) attached to an IV pole using adjustable bracket that allows the height of the assembly to be adjusted. A laser level is attached to the transducer holder (*B*), allowing the height of the transducers to be matched to markings on the patient. With the patient seated and stationary on the ergometer, a horizontal mark is made at the level of the fourth anterior intercostal space and a vertical mark is made along the mid-axillary line (*C*); this line is used to adjust the height of the transducers when the patient is supine. The laser level is used to place a horizontal mark on the patient's back at the same height as the horizontal axillary line (*D*); this line is used to adjust the height of the transducers when the patient is upright on the ergometer or in the chair. Tape is placed on the IV pole to allow for rapid leveling of the transducers when the patient is exercising on the ergometer (*upper tape line*) or resting in the chair (*lower tape line*) (*E*). Once the patient is supine on the cath table, the transducer height is adjusted to match the previously drawn mid-axillary line (*F*).

have also shown that the pulmonary vascular resistance measured in the upright position (both at rest and during exercise) exceeds measures in the supine position by 10%.[24] Such differences between supine and upright hemodynamics can be significant to the point that they impact diagnosis. For example, Rao and colleagues have shown how an upright iCPET is capable of reclassifying heart failure with preserved ejection fraction (diagnosed by supine iCPET) to cardiac preload failure.[25] Regardless of the body position that is

chosen for iCPET, accurate analysis requires that the team performing the study is familiar with normal hemodynamic ranges for the testing position.

Cardiac Output Measurement

CO measurement is an essential part of the iCPET. The gold standard for determination is the direct Fick principle, which requires placement of a radial arterial catheter to measure SaO_2.[19] The thermodilution is considered a reliable alternative method for measuring CO at rest and during exercise[19] (though it is recommended that more than one measurement be performed, which can be challenging during an iCPET). Risbano and colleagues recently demonstrated that calculation of CO with reliance upon SpO_2 by a pulse oximeter, rather than SaO_2, for calculation of CO can result in misclassification of pulmonary hypertension in certain populations.[26]

Waveform Interpretation and Respiratory Swings

Interpretation of hemodynamic waveforms during exercise can be challenging, and experts continue to debate the pros and cons of using computer-generated mean versus end-expiratory hemodynamic measurements.[19] This important topic is discussed in more detail in Sarma's contribution to this volume.

Need for Supplemental Oxygen During Invasive Cardiopulmonary Exercise Test

If patients require the use of supplemental oxygen during an iCPET, it is recommended that a nondiffusing collection bag (Douglas bag) that is large enough to meet the subject's volume requirements at maximum exercise be added to the system. The specific Fio_2 used may need to be updated in the metabolic cart diagnostic software to assure accuracy of the results.

SUMMARY

While an iCPET study is both complex and initially intimidating from a program building perspective, the information gained through a high-quality study can often add critical information to the evaluation of patients with a wide (and growing) range of conditions. It is our hope that this article demystifies the process by which an iCPET is set up and performed. It is important to note that a successful iCPET study requires more than just the equipment and techniques discussed in this article. As discussed in the companion piece in this series, "How to Start an Invasive Cardiopulmonary Exercise Testing Program: A Comprehensive and Practical Guide" by Michael Risbano, an iCPET is more of a program than a stand-alone test. Given this, we recommend that centers aspiring to start an iCPET program visit one or more established program(s) in order to expand upon the information presented in this article and, in doing so, develop a protocol that meets their particular needs and draws upon their strengths.

CLINICS CARE POINTS

- A high-quality invasive cardiopulmonary exercise test (iCPET) provides essential data regarding the causes of exercise intolerance that cannot be obtained through other testing modalities.
- Performing and interpreting an iCPET should be undertaken using a multidisciplinary team–based approach.
- Essential decisions regarding how to address key issues, such as body position during exercise, zeroing of the PA catheter, measurement of cardiac output, and safety precautions during testing must be made early in the development of a center-specific iCPET protocol.
- Performing a high-quality iCPET starts with obtaining an iCPET protocol (such as the one included in this article), visiting established iCPET centers to observe multiple studies and modification of the protocol fit the needs and draws upon center-specific strengths.

ACKNOWLEDGMENTS

The authors would like to thank Dr Michael Risbano, who kindly contributed his iCPET protocol from the University of Pittsburgh Advanced Cardiopulmonary Exercise Testing Program.

DISCLOSURE

S.H. Visovatti has served as a consultant for United Therapeutics. Dr B.A. Maron reports receiving personal fees from Actelion Pharmaceuticals, personal fees from Tenax, personal fees from Regeneron, and grants from Deerfield Company.

REFERENCES

1. Rischard BAB FP. Tool sof the trade: how do you perform and interpret an exercise test? Advances in Pulmonary Hypertension 2019;18(No 2):47–55.
2. American Thoracic S, American College of Chest P. ATS/ACCP Statement on cardiopulmonary exercise testing. Am J Respir Crit Care Med 2003;167(2):211–77.
3. Berry NC, Manyoo A, Oldham WM, et al. Protocol for exercise hemodynamic assessment: performing an invasive cardiopulmonary exercise test in clinical practice. Pulm Circ 2015;5(4):610–8.
4. Maron BA, Cockrill BA, Waxman AB, et al. The invasive cardiopulmonary exercise test. Circulation 2013;127(10):1157–64.

5. Allen J. Interpreting the cardiopulmonary exercise test. Available at: https://hospitalmedicaldirector.com/interpreting-the-cardiopulmonary-exercise-test/.

6. Tang WHW, Wilcox JD, Jacob MS, et al. Comprehensive diagnostic evaluation of cardiovascular physiology in patients with pulmonary vascular disease: insights from the PVDOMICS program. Circ Heart Fail 2020;13(3):e006363.

7. Joseph P, Arevalo C, Oliveira RKF, et al. Insights from invasive cardiopulmonary exercise testing of patients with myalgic encephalomyelitis/chronic fatigue syndrome. Chest 2021;160(2):642–51.

8. Singh I, Joseph P, Heerdt PM, et al. Persistent exertional intolerance after COVID-19: insights from invasive cardiopulmonary exercise testing. Chest 2022; 161(1):54–63.

9. Risbano MGKCRDDGK C, Campedelli L, Yoney K, et al. Invasive cardiopulmonary exercise testing identifies distinct physiologic endotypes in postacute sequelae of SARS-CoV-2 infection. Chest Pulmonary 2023;1(3).

10. Kahn PA, Joseph P, Heerdt PM, et al. Differential cardiopulmonary haemodynamic phenotypes in PASC-related exercise intolerance. ERJ Open Res 2024;10(1).

11. Singh I, Leitner BP, Wang Y, et al. Proteomic profiling demonstrates inflammatory and endotheliopathy signatures associated with impaired cardiopulmonary exercise hemodynamic profile in Post Acute Sequelae of SARS-CoV-2 infection (PASC) syndrome. Pulm Circ 2023;13(2):e12220.

12. Oldham WM, Oliveira RKF, Wang RS, et al. Network analysis to risk stratify patients with exercise intolerance. Circ Res 2018;122(6):864–76.

13. Joseph P, Pari R, Miller S, et al. Neurovascular dysregulation and acute exercise intolerance in myalgic encephalomyelitis/chronic fatigue syndrome: a randomized, placebo-controlled trial of pyridostigmine. Chest 2022;162(5):1116–26.

14. Jain CC, Borlaug BA. Performance and interpretation of invasive hemodynamic exercise testing. Chest 2020;158(5):2119–29.

15. Ward K. Wasserman & Whipp's principles of exercise testing and interpretation. 6th edition. Wolters Kluwer. Lippincott Williams & Wilkins; 2020.

16. Huang W, Resch S, Oliveira RK, et al. Invasive cardiopulmonary exercise testing in the evaluation of unexplained dyspnea: insights from a multidisciplinary dyspnea center. Eur J Prev Cardiol 2017; 24(11):1190–9.

17. Chambers DJ, Wisely NA. Cardiopulmonary exercise testing-a beginner's guide to the nine-panel plot. BJA Educ 2019;19(5):158–64.

18. Glaab T, Taube C. Practical guide to cardiopulmonary exercise testing in adults. Respir Res 2022; 23(1):9.

19. Kovacs G, Herve P, Barbera JA, et al. An official European Respiratory Society statement: pulmonary haemodynamics during exercise. Eur Respir J 2017;50(5).

20. Humbert M, Kovacs G, Hoeper MM, et al. ESC/ERS Guidelines for the diagnosis and treatment of pulmonary hypertension. Eur Heart J 2022;43(38):3618–731.

21. Sandoval Y, Bell MR, Gulati R. Transradial artery access complications. Circ Cardiovasc Interv 2019; 12(11):e007386.

22. Ibe T, Wada H, Sakakura K, et al. Right ventricular stroke work index. Int Heart J 2018;59(5):1047–51.

23. Ferguson C, Girardi M, DeCato TW. Supine vs upright exercise: far-reaching implications for invasive cardiopulmonary exercise test interpretation. Chest 2024;165(5):1046–8.

24. Berlier C, Saxer S, Lichtblau M, et al. Influence of upright versus supine position on resting and exercise hemodynamics in patients assessed for pulmonary hypertension. J Am Heart Assoc 2022;11(4): e023839.

25. Rao VN, Kelsey MD, Blazing MA, et al. Unexplained dyspnea on exertion: the difference the right test can make. Circ Heart Fail 2022;15(2):e008982.

26. Campedelli L, Nouraie SM, Risbano MG. Non-arterial line cardiac output calculation misclassifies exercise pulmonary hypertension and increases risk of data loss particularly in black, Scleroderma, and Raynaud's patients during invasive exercise testing. Eur Respir J 2024. https://doi.org/10.1183/13993003.02232-2023.

How to Start an Invasive Cardiopulmonary Exercise Testing Program
A Comprehensive and Practical Guide

Michael G. Risbano, MD, MA[a,b,c,*]

KEYWORDS

- Exercise testing • iCPET • Invasive cardiopulmonary exercise testing • Business plan
- Starting a program • Exercise pulmonary hypertension

KEY POINTS

- Invasive Cardiopulmonary Exercise Testing (iCPET) Program Development: This manuscript serves as a comprehensive guide to establishing an iCPET program, detailing the necessary steps from conceptualization to implementation.
- Multidisciplinary Approach: Emphasizes the importance of collaboration across cardiology and pulmonary divisions to successfully integrate and manage iCPET services within a health care setting.
- Business and Operational Considerations: Discusses the creation of a robust business plan, including stakeholder engagement, financial planning, and strategic marketing to ensure the sustainability and growth of the iCPET program.

INTRODUCTION

Invasive cardiopulmonary exercise testing (iCPET) is a harmonious union of breath-by-breath physiologic evaluation with cardiopulmonary hemodynamics during exercise, producing a comprehensive assessment of individual exercise capacity and limitations. iCPET has become a vital clinical and research instrument to assess and manage a variety of cardiovascular and respiratory conditions. iCPET is typically performed at academic centers and requires a significant infrastructure to support and develop the program. This manuscript is a personal accounting of my efforts to develop the University of Pittsburgh Medical Center (UPMC) iCPET program. As I wrote this article, I reflected on the long hours and hard work to move this program forward. I, like other physicians, am no stranger to working long hours. But starting and leading a program de novo was a new experience for me. I fortunately had the support of our Cardiology and Pulmonary/Critical Care administrations and was equipped with vital resources. Though supported, I did encounter many hardships. During the early years of the program, I carried a perpetual and haunting worry that the

[a] Division of Pulmonary, Allergy, and Critical Care Medicine, Department of Medicine, Post-COVID Recovery Clinic, University of Pittsburgh School of Medicine and UPMC, Pittsburgh, PA, USA; [b] Center for Pulmonary Vascular Biology and Medicine, Pittsburgh Heart, Lung, Blood Vascular Medicine Institute, University of Pittsburgh School of Medicine and UPMC, Pittsburgh, PA, USA; [c] Division of Pulmonary, Allergy, Critical Care and Sleep Medicine, Department of Medicine, Vascular Medicine Institute, University of Pittsburgh Medical Center, Montefiore Hospital, NW 628, 3459 Fifth Avenue, Pittsburgh, PA 15213, USA
* Division of Pulmonary, Allergy, Critical Care and Sleep Medicine, Department of Medicine, Vascular Medicine Institute, University of Pittsburgh Medical Center, Montefiore Hospital, NW 628, 3459 Fifth Avenue, Pittsburgh, PA 15213.
E-mail address: risbanomg@upmc.edu

Heart Failure Clin 21 (2025) 93–109
https://doi.org/10.1016/j.hfc.2024.06.012
1551-7136/25/© 2024 Elsevier Inc. All rights are reserved, including those for text and data mining, AI training, and similar technologies.

iCPET program would not be successful and could be removed from my leadership—at any time.

Those Were Challenging Days. Was It Worth It?

This manuscript is intended to be a comprehensive and personal guide outlining in detail the process of establishing an iCPET program. I will address the following topics in this manuscript: stakeholder engagement, the pros and cons of starting an iCPET program, the composition of the necessary team, the development of a robust business plan, and practical steps for setting up and running the program effectively.

MY PATH TO EXERCISE PHYSIOLOGY

Each iCPET program will most likely have a different origin, different rationale for its creation, as well as different stakeholders. I am providing personal background about my experience as this directly influenced the growth and development of the UPMC iCPET program.

I initially learned the art of right heart catheterizations at the University of Colorado during my Pulmonary Sciences and Critical Care Fellowship as a pulmonary hypertension trainee. On September 1, 2010, I was recruited to the Division of Pulmonary, Allergy, and Critical Care Medicine at UPMC. As part of my recruitment, I ensured that I had privileges to perform right heart catheterizations in the cath laboratory at UPMC. From 2010 to 2016, I developed a growing interest in exercise hemodynamics, publishing several manuscripts utilizing supine exercise right heart catheterization as a research platform.[1–3]

In 2015, the leadership of the pulmonary vascular program expressed interest in developing an iCPET program. I saw this as an opportunity and took the lead in establishing the program. There was a slight challenge, however: I was a pulmonologist planning to lead a cardiology-funded program. Despite this, the Cardiology and Pulmonary Divisions at UPMC had a history of cooperative work in the pulmonary vascular space. The primary challenges we faced were related to funding and ownership of this emerging program.

It was made clear that to run the iCPET program, I needed to develop a business plan, identify and engage with key stakeholders, and establish milestones and deliverables. These were all terms and concepts I was not immediately familiar with. Fortunately, I obtained a business plan blueprint from an established iCPET program. Although my final business plan deviated significantly from this initial version, it provided a valuable starting point, raising questions and programmatic concerns I had not considered.

This process began in October 2016. I met with key stakeholders from the Divisions of Cardiology and Pulmonary, where I presented my vision, timeline, and milestones. **Table 1** shows the proposed and actual timelines for the iCPET program.

WHERE DO YOU BEGIN?

It starts with the idea that you want to test physiologic principles beyond standard CPET. There are many reasons to start an iCPET program. There are also many reasons not to start an iCPET program. Think about your vision for the program: the type of services you plan to provide; meaningful career and programmatic milestones; and the levels of discomfort you are willing to deal with throughout this process.

PRE-CONSIDERATIONS

The first question you should ask yourself is, "Why?" Why are you starting an iCPET program? It might be your idea, or it could be driven by the leadership in your division. But why start an iCPET program? Are you interested in the clinical investigation of exercise physiology (EP) and hemodynamics? Do you want to employ physiologic findings as part of a research career? Are you committed to obtaining funding for the program? Are you prepared to spend a significant amount of time establishing, maintaining, and worrying about the program? Are you willing to devote considerable time to performing and interpreting iCPET studies?

If you want to run the program correctly, this is the reality you will face. While there are ways to build a team to delegate tasks and support these efforts, this requires additional funding and time to actively manage a team. If you want the program to run smoothly and correctly, you need to take a hands-on approach.

CONSIDERATIONS FOR DEVELOPING AN INVASIVE CARDIOPULMONARY EXERCISE TESTING PROGRAM

Before committing to starting a program, think about the positives and negatives of establishing an iCPET program. Below are some considerations.

Pros

1. *Enhanced diagnostic accuracy.* iCPET provides detailed insights into cardiac and pulmonary function under stress, facilitating precise diagnosis.
2. *Tailored treatment plans.* The data gleaned from iCPET enable the formulation of personalized

Table 1
My proposed and actual timeline in establishing the iCPET Program at UPMC

Proposed Date	Actual Date	Event
September 15–18th 2016	September 15–18th 2016	CHEST CPET program education, Chicago, Illinois
September–November 2016	September 26, 2017	Planning and education Visit to Brigham and Women's Investigate iCPET equipment needed
October–December 2016	May 12, 2017	Obtain iCPET equipment Identify staff to assist in performance of iCPET
December 2016	May 25, 2017	Practice testing and education of staff Increase awareness of the program and recruitment through education, talks, presentations
January 2017	June 7, 2017	Perform the first iCPET study Continue to increase awareness of the program and recruitment through education, talks, presentations
April 2017	July 2017	Anticipated time that 2 iCPET can be performed per day.

treatment strategies based on individual patient responses.

3. *Research opportunities.* iCPET programs contribute to ongoing research endeavors, fostering advancements in cardiovascular and pulmonary medicine.
4. *The pure joy of engaging with physiology.* Physiology does not lie; it is the closest to the truth that one can encounter. Sometimes interpretations of the data may be incorrect, but physiology is always true.

Cons

1. *Invasive nature.* The inherent risks associated with invasive procedures necessitate a meticulous risk-benefit analysis.
2. *Resource intensive.* iCPET programs demand specialized equipment, trained personnel, and dedicated facilities. These necessary resources result in higher initial costs, as well as ongoing operational costs to maintain the program.
3. *Time commitment.* These studies are a large time commitment. Each study takes 1.5 hours to 2 hours to perform by a single operator with a team. This does not include the time for informed consent, explaining the results of the studies, collecting the data, and then contacting referring physicians and patients. Each study could require a 4–5-h time investment.
4. *Poor relative value units (RVU) for the amount of work performed.* If you are looking to get rich performing iCPETs, forget it. The financial

reimbursement is low relative to the time spent executing these studies and running a program. It is unlikely that an iCPET program would be viable in a non-academic setting. Our break-even point is 2 studies per day; so greater than or equal to 3 studies per day may result in positive revenue. Is it feasible to perform more studies than your identified breakeven point? **Table 2** shows common CPT codes charged for an iCPET study.

Box 1 includes questions to think about before beginning an iCPET Program.

Table 2
Procedures performed during iCPET studies

Procedure	CPT Code
Pulmonary Stress Complex	94.621
Right Heart Catheterization	93.451
Arterial Line Insertion with Sampling	36.620
Blood Gas with Saturations (arterial and pulmonary artery) with lactate up to 16+ total	82.803
Ultrasound x 2	76.937
Spirometry	94.010

Radial and pulmonary arterial blood gases are performed at rest seated, freewheel, stage 1, 2, 3, 4, 5, and post exercise for a total of 16 gases. Each stage of exercise is 2 minutes, therefore these gases are run every 2 minutes during exercise.

Box 1
Important clinical questions to ask prior to starting an iCPET program

Questions to ask yourself prior to starting an iC-PET program.

Financial

- What is the anticipated and expected patient volume through this program?
- Is this a sustainable volume to cover the costs of running the program?
- What is the expected reimbursement from these procedures?
- Is there a commitment from your division Chief or Chair of Medicine to continue the program even at a financial loss? Access to an iCPET program at a tertiary or quaternary care center may be necessary to provide care to medically complex patients even at a financial loss.
- Who is paying for the initial investment of equipment, consumed supplies, maintenance, and new equipment as the program ages?
- Are there institutional funds or grants available to help cover the costs of the program?
- How will you be reimbursed for your efforts?
- Do the RVUs generated from your efforts go to your Division? Do you get the RVU credit?
- Who retains the institutional RVU billing? Is there sharing between different divisions if this is a joint program (i.e. between pulmonary and cardiology)?

Stakeholders

- Who are the stakeholders in your program, or division?
- Do you have the support of your division to start a program?
- Who will be an essential part of the team to help ensure your goals?
- What is the division expecting from your program-clinically, financially, research-wise?
- Is there anyone who will be particularly threatened by the initiation of an iCPET program?
- Is there anyone in the institution who would flat-out oppose the start of an iCPET program?
- How do you plan to resolve areas of potential conflict?
- Are you leading this program on your own, or will you have a partner?
- Is there another local iCPET program? Are you in direct competition for patients?

Location, location, location

- Where will the studies be performed?
- Will the RHC and arterial line be placed in the cath laboratory, and the exercise portion occurs in a separate exercise room, or will both procedures be performed in the same room as we do at UPMC?
- Do you have a room and staff guaranteed for the entire day?
- What is the cath laboratory patient volume? What would happen if you tie up a room for half of a day or the entire day?
- Will an iCPET study create a bottleneck in the cath laboratory workflow? How will you negotiate this with the cath laboratory? What concessions are you willing to make?
- If you cannot perform your studies at the main hospital at your center, is there a peripheral site that may welcome the volume of patients that you would bring? Although this may not be as prestigious, a welcoming site to perform iCPET with available resources is more valuable than you may think. Know your worth but know your limitations.

Clinical staffing

- What staff do you need in order to perform these studies correctly?
- Can you hire and pay for the staffing required? Or will certain staff members be on loan from other departments?
- Who will manage the metabolic cart? An exercise physiologist, respiratory therapist, or another staff member?
- What are the minimal number of cath laboratory members that you need? Some institutions have a policy that requires 3 cath laboratory staff per room (techs and nurses).

Research

- Do you plan on utilizing the data generated for research purposes?
- Do you need to hire someone to manage your iCPET database?
- What platform will you use for the database? From personal experience Microsoft excel sheets and paper charts do not suffice.
- What assistance do you have to collect blood samples and transport them to the research lab?
- Who will process the research blood samples?
- Who will store, label and manage the research blood samples?
- Have you set up an IRB to collect these samples? Do you have an informed consent process?

- Do you need a study coordinator and regulatory personnel to assist with this process?
- Is there grant money available to facilitate your research goals?

Your iCPET program

- Will the program operate independently, or will it be part of a larger clinical program such as an exercise intolerance or dyspnea program?
- What is the referral process to the iCPET program?
- Who will schedule these patients for you?
- How do you plan on keeping tack of the referrals and ensuring they are properly scheduled?
- How will you advertise the program?
- What is the patient population are you targeting?
- Will an iCPET be performed to evaluate a particular disease state (that is, chronic pulmonary embolism, or HFpEF) or will you perform iCPET on subjects referred for undifferentiated exercise intolerance/dyspnea on exertion?
- What work-up is required prior to ordering an iCPET study?
- Are there any patients that you would not feel comfortable performing an exercise study on?
- What volume can you handle? How many studies do you plan on performing in 1 day?
- How many days of week do you plan on performing these studies?
- What is your goal number of studies to perform in 1 year?
- How will you notify the referring physician, and the patient about the results?
- How will you handle any potential complications due to this procedure?
- How does follow-up occur after the procedure?
- Who prescribes medications, or orders the subsequent testing after the iCPET test?
- Will you see all patients in clinic prior to testing, or are you comfortable performing only the procedure without a pre-existing clinical relationship?

DEVELOP A BUSINESS PLAN

Creating a business plan is essential for clearly outlining your vision for the program and its needs.

This plan will help both you and the stakeholders understand what is required to establish and sustain the program. Think of yourself as a small business owner starting a new venture. You need to produce a value-added product (diagnostic testing in the form of iCPET) that others (referring physicians) will want to utilize.

To successfully launch the program, you need to.

1. Brand the Program: Choose a name that reflects the essence of your program. Clearly state your mission and vision to guide its development.
2. Identify a Target Population: Determine the specific group of patients you intend to study and serve.
3. Develop a Referral Network: Build relationships with referring physicians who can send patients your way.
4. Engage a Marketing Team: Work with marketing professionals to promote your program effectively.
5. Create a Financial Plan: Develop a financial strategy to cover the costs of the program.

While business plans can be customized to fit specific needs, some key considerations include the following.

Name Your Program

Naming your program may seem straightforward but can be challenging. How do you want to communicate the intent and purpose of your program in as few, yet descriptive, words as possible? I initially took a simple and non-creative approach, naming it the UPMC iCPET Program. However, our media department felt that "invasive" was too "invasive" and may have a negative connotation, so the name was subsequently refined to the UPMC Advanced Cardiopulmonary Exercise Testing (aCPET) Program. While not very creative, the name effectively conveys the program's function.

Create a Mission Statement

What is the goal and purpose of your iCPET Program? Reflecting on my initial mission statement, I realize my goals have shifted. Initially, it read: "The Center for Invasive Cardiopulmonary Exercise Testing will provide multidisciplinary and comprehensive iCPET for clinical and research purposes to study and diagnose abnormal pulmonary vascular responses to exercise." Today, the mission statement is: "The aCPET Program provides comprehensive iCPET for clinical and research purposes to offer diagnostic and prognostic information for patients presenting with dyspnea on exertion and/or exercise intolerance."

The program has expanded beyond pulmonary vascular disease and has become an essential next step for referring physicians when testing has been inconclusive or unable to identify the causes of exercise intolerance.

Identify Your Vision for the Program

My initial vision for the program was based on a 3-tiered approach: (1) Clinical Investigation, (2) Research, and (3) Funding. I later changed the third pillar to Education, particularly for fellows-in-training.

- *Clinical Investigation*: The iCPET program will perform resting and exercise hemodynamics coupled with arterial blood gas measurements and cardiopulmonary exercise testing to investigate the cardiopulmonary physiologic response to exercise as a stressor.
- *Research*: Research will be a strong component of this program. We will use clinical investigations to identify specific disease phenotypes for research studies. All subjects undergoing iCPET will be consented to collect clinical data and biological samples for research purposes.
- *Funding*: Efforts will be made to obtain federal and institutional support. Funding may also come from partnerships with other investigators interested in using iCPET as a diagnostic or research tool.
- *Education*: The aCPET program will provide pulmonary and cardiovascular medicine fellows-in-training an opportunity to learn the physiologic basis of cardiopulmonary diseases through first-hand exposure to gas exchange and hemodynamic parameters measured during iCPET studies.

Identify Your Referral Base

Referrals will be generated from physicians interested in answering EP-based questions. The referral base for the iCPET Program will include subspecialists from the fields of cardiology, pulmonology, rheumatology, and primary care. We have also received referrals from pediatrics for adult patients with congenital heart disease, or possible mitochondrial myopathy.

Establish Indications for Invasive Cardiopulmonary Exercise Testing and Patient Populations

Overall, 2 types of patient populations are referred for an iCPET study. (1) Undifferentiated dyspnea on exertion and/or exercise intolerance where initial diagnostic testing has been unrevealing[4–8]; and (2) Patients with known or suspected disease states including but not limited to post-pulmonary embolism, heart failure, parenchymal lung disease, scleroderma, pulmonary vascular disease, dysautonomia, or more recently long-coronavirus disease (COVID).[9] The goal of iCPET is to identify physiologic disturbances that may be due to one of the following, or potentially overlapping diagnoses: pulmonary vascular disease (pulmonary arterial hypertension, exercise pulmonary hypertension, chronic pulmonary embolism),[1,3,10–18] left-sided heart disease (heart failure with preserved or reduced ejection fraction, valvular disease),[19–22] ventilatory limitation (chronic obstructive pulmonary disease [COPD], interstitial lung disease, asthma),[23] decreased oxygen extraction (mitochondrial myopathy),[10,24] neurovascular dysfunction (pre-load insufficiency)[25,26] or deconditioning.

Anticipate the Impact of an Invasive Cardiopulmonary Exercise Testing Program**

Consider the impact your iCPET program will have on the institution. Which patient populations will benefit from the program (see above), and what will referring physicians gain from sending their patients for these studies? Understanding these aspects is essential to garnering support from stakeholders.

Realistically Estimate the Number of Studies to Be Performed**

We estimated that the number of iCPET studies performed in 1 year would be similar to the number of exercise right heart catheterizations conducted annually. We used data from the previous 5 years to create this estimate. Additionally, we considered the number of patients diagnosed with exercise pulmonary hypertension, heart failure with preserved ejection fraction (HFpEF), and normal findings to understand the types of diagnoses we might encounter.

However, iCPET can identify a broader range of conditions beyond cardiovascular and pulmonary vascular diseases, thus expanding the types of diagnoses our program can address. Based on my clinical workload, we anticipated that performing 2 iCPET studies per day could potentially result in 96 iCPET studies per year.

Determine How Invasive Cardiopulmonary Exercise Testing Equipment Will be Purchased

Metabolic carts are expensive, and securing funding for them is crucial. Consider the following questions.

- Is your division willing to pay for the equipment? If so, what do they expect in return?
- Will the division collect institutional RVUs to recuperate the cost?

- Are they prepared to run the program at a financial deficit?
- Will you need to reimburse the cost of the metabolic carts?

Understanding how many studies you plan on performing and identifying the revenue flow is important. You will need to present this information to the key stakeholders to secure their support and funding.

WHO ARE THE KEY STAKEHOLDERS?

Stakeholders are simply anyone interested in ensuring the success of the iCPET program, or who would incur an increased workload because of the downstream effort created by the program. Stakeholders may also include other exercise testing programs that may compete for similar resources or patients. There may be institutional variability, but in general key stakeholders may include the following:

Division leadership–include the academic Division Chief, and the Clinical Chief if the program is structured in this manner as it is at the University of Pittsburgh. Most cardiopulmonary exercise testing programs are housed within either the Pulmonary Division or Cardiovascular Medicine Division. Specific upfront topics to discuss with leadership include.

- The availability of funding to purchase expensive equipment.
- An academic stipend for the iCPET program leadership.
- Funding for iCPET staff, including those performing administrative services.
- Determination of revenue flow to recuperate investment into the program.
- Potential programmatic cost sharing between interested divisions, and distribution of RVUs to the physician performing these studies. For example, if the iCPET studies are performed in the cardiac cath laboratory by a pulmonologist, will the associated costs and revenue collection be shared between the Pulmonary and Cardiovascular Medicine Divisions?
- Establishment of referral and outreach initiatives.
- Development of an iCPET research program. Specific topics include dedicated resources for blood sample collection, processing and storage, as well as the establishment of a database.

CARDIOPULMONARY EXERCISE TESTING DIRECTOR

Institutions with active CPET programs may perceive an iCPET program as competition. It is crucial to meet with the CPET Program Director to identify the synergy between the 2 diagnostic modalities. For instance, our iCPET program often receives referrals for patients who have undergone a non-invasive CPET study and require further evaluation for conditions such as pulmonary vascular disease, cardiac disease including HFpEF, or dysautonomia.

Key items to discuss include.

- Identifying the limitations of non-invasive exercise testing and highlighting how iCPET serves as a valuable, complementary diagnostic modality. iCPET can identify conditions that non-invasive CPET cannot, such as preload insufficiency, exercise pulmonary hypertension, HFpEF, and decreased peripheral oxygen extraction.
- Coordinating the workflow between the CPET and iCPET programs.
- Establishing the logistics of the referral process.
- Determining the patient populations and disease states that may benefit from iCPET.

Cardiac Catheterization Laboratory Director

If iCPET studies are to be performed in the cardiac cath laboratory, a meeting with the physician and nursing cath laboratory directors, as well as hospital administrative leadership, is essential. Key items to discuss include.

- *Identification of Physical Space*: Determine the available physical space for performing studies and the appropriate area for storing CPET equipment and the bicycle ergometer.
- Scheduling: Select the days of the week that studies can be performed.
- *Staffing Requirements*: Determine the number of staff required to perform the study, including nurses and cath laboratory technicians.
- *Workflow*: Establish the proper workflow from patient admission to discharge.

Additionally, if the equipment is housed in the cardiac cath laboratory, a discussion with Biomedical Engineers will be necessary to ensure the proper functioning and calibration of the equipment used during iCPET. It is also crucial to identify administrative staff responsible for scheduling, handling associated paperwork, study authorizations, and communication with patients and referring physicians.

These studies are time and labor-intensive from the start of the study to cleaning the room. In a busy cardiac cath laboratory, rapid turnover is necessary, and iCPET studies can slow down the work process. Therefore, it is important to discuss the amount of cath laboratory time available for each iCPET study on a given day. Additionally, determine if there will be time to extract data from the metabolic cart computer immediately after the study in the cath laboratory or if the data need to be collected at another time.

Exercise Physiology Director

An experienced EP team is a critical component of a safe, high-quality iCPET study. While most exercise physiologists may initially have limited experience with invasive CPET, many core aspects are similar to non-invasive CPET. Early discussions with the EP Director are essential for the successful development of an iCPET program. Key items to discuss include.

- *Selection of Equipment*: Choose the metabolic cart and ergometer best suited for iCPET studies.
- *Safety Protocols*: Develop comprehensive safety protocols for testing.
- *Scheduling Coordination*: Coordinate schedules, considering that most EPs have responsibilities in non-invasive CPET and cardiac stress testing laboratories. Scheduling iCPET studies must account for the busy EP schedule.

ABG Lab Director

A single iCPET study requires processing a significant number of blood gases over a short period. Depending on the study duration and frequency of blood gas draws, 12 to over 20 blood gases may be collected. Institutions may have different departments processing blood gases. For example, at UPMC Presbyterian, blood gases were processed at the clinical laboratory within the Department of Pathology. At the Shadyside Hospital, blood gases were processed in the ABG lab run by the Respiratory Department. In some systems, the cath laboratory has a dedicated blood gas machine, significantly shortening the turnaround time for sample processing but requiring certified cath laboratory personnel to operate the machine during iCPET studies. Key items to discuss include.

- *Laboratory Capacity*: Assess the laboratory's capacity to process large numbers of blood gases quickly.
- *Sample Processing*: Determine whether all blood gas samples should be sent to the laboratory at once or in smaller batches.
- *Sample Collection and Transportation Protocol*: Develop a protocol for sample collection and transportation, including whether samples should be placed on ice and whether

they should be hand-delivered or sent through a tube system (the latter is generally not recommended).

BUILD A TEAM

The following is the list of staffing that I require to maintain the iCPET Program.

- Exercise physiologist, 20% effort, 1 day/week. I have access to 2 staff members that alternate study days. 1 exercise physiologist's time is covered through the Department of Cardiac Rehabilitation and the other I have recently hired with grant funds.
- 2 Cath laboratory nurses (provided by the Cath laboratory), 20% effort, 1 day/week covered by cath laboratory payroll.
- 1 Cath laboratory tech (provided by the Cath laboratory), 20% effort, 1 day/week covered by cath laboratory payroll.
- Data base manager, 20% effort. Partial effort covered by an internal grant.
- Post-Doctoral Fellow, 100% effort, 5 days/week. Effort covered by an internal grant.
- Clinic nurse (Pulmonary Hypertension Clinic Nurse)
- Cath laboratory scheduler, covered by the cath laboratory payroll.
- Research Coordinator, who also performs regulatory work for the program. Partial effort covered by the Shadyside Foundation Grant.
- 1 Respiratory therapist to run blood gases for cases twice a day, effort covered by the Department of Respiratory Therapy.
- Biomedical engineers, provided by the hospital.
- iCPET Director (1 full day per week)

The team of cath laboratory nurses and techs varies daily depending on assignments. Since the staff cycles through the cath laboratory, everyone stays familiar with the iCPET protocol. You may not always have the same staff members assigned to your laboratory each week, which can be frustrating if you work better with some team members than others. The key is to ensure that all staff members rotating through the laboratory remain appropriately trained. Keep calm, delegate tasks, lead effectively, and work with the available staff. They are essential to ensuring your cases go as smoothly as possible.

Visit an Invasive Cardiopulmonary Exercise Testing Program

While it is possible to develop an iCPET program by reading resources, scouring the internet, and speaking with program leaders at other sites, nothing can replace an in-person visit to see an iCPET program in action. Each site will have a different approach and workflow, consisting of team members with various skill sets. The study may be performed in different clinical settings; for example, some programs conduct the resting portion in the cath laboratory and then transfer the patient to a dedicated room for the exercise portion.

It is often the small, nuanced factors that get overlooked when planning a program, which can result in bottlenecks if not addressed upfront. The bane of medical practice is not knowing what you do not know. We have hosted individuals interested in developing an iCPET program and welcome visitors to observe our process firsthand.

INVASIVE CARDIOPULMONARY EXERCISE TESTING DEFINED

Currently, there are no established guidelines or consensus from professional societies regarding the procedural components required an iCPET study.[8,27] Some programs consider an right heart catheterization (RHC) with a metabolic cart but no arterial line as an iCPET study, while others consider arterial line as an essential component of an iCPET study. We believe that an RHC with a metabolic cart and arterial line should be considered the gold standard for exercise testing. The absence of an arterial line and blood gas samples results in inaccurate measurement of O_2 saturations, as well as data loss during exercise, particularly in black patients and those with scleroderma and/or Raynaud's.[28] Additonally, the Fick cardiac output calculation without arterial blood samples is inaccurate, leading to misclassification of pre- and post-capillary exercise pulmonary hypertension (ePH).[28] Overall, placing a temporary radial arterial line in the outpatient setting is considered to be low risk for the patient.

We advocate for the use of an upright ergometer to assess exercise physiology (EP). While pulmonary vascular resistance measured in the upright position may closely correlate with supine exercise assessments,[29] conditions such as preload insufficiency require an upright position for detection.[30] Supine positioning may therefore miss diagnoses in certain pathologic disease states and may be uncomfortable for patients with orthopnea, abdominal obesity, or for elderly patients. Semi-recumbent exercise may also not fully reflect hemodynamics in the upright position, and the upright position is associated with achieving higher peak oxygen consumption compared to the semi-recumbent position.[31,32] Ultimately, the iCPET program director and institution must decide on the most feasible

and effective exercise methodology, considering the clinical population under investigation.

DEVELOP YOUR WORKFLOW IN ADVANCE

Although it may be difficult to envision your workflow before starting a program, discuss your options with stakeholders to develop the best execution plan. Take time to train the staff before performing any studies. Set up meetings with team members, prepare the room with the necessary equipment, and conduct several dry run studies with a staff member playing the role of the patient. These practice sessions help establish expectations and identify areas of weakness that need to be addressed.

Box 2 outlines our typical workflow for an iCPET study, from the initial referral to the completion of the study. When starting an iCPET program, there may be a tendency to experiment with different methods, leading to variations in the study process and potential confusion among staff. Once you establish an effective workflow, ensure that each study is performed consistently. Today, we follow the same procedure for every study, which helps maintain consistency and reduces mistakes, even when different staff members rotate into the cath laboratory.

OUR INVASIVE CARDIOPULMONARY EXERCISE TESTING PROCEDURE

Our procedural approach is as follows: We typically begin by placing place a 20-gauge radial arterial catheter (Arrow, Morrisville NC, USA) into the non-dominant radial artery under ultrasound guidance. Then a 7.5 Fr pulmonary artery (PA) quadruple lumen VIP catheter (Edwards Lifesciences, Irvine, CA, USA) is placed through an 8F introducer sheath into the right internal jugular vein under ultrasound and fluoroscopic guidance. A right heart catheterization is performed in the supine position. Zero reference level is mid-axillary when supine.[33] We average hemodynamic values over 3 to 4 respiratory cycles. Standard hemodynamic values are collected including right atrium, right ventricle, PA, pulmonary artery wedge (PW) and cardiac output by indirect Fick and thermodilution (see **Box 2**).

Patients are then directed to perform a symptom-limited incremental peak exercise study on an upright cycle ergometer (Lode, Ultima CPX, MGC Diagnostics, St. Paul, MN, USA) with a continuous ramp protocol ranging from 5 W/minute to 20 W/minute while maintaining 55 rpm to 65 rpm. We encouraged patients to exercise to a maximal goal respiratory exchange ratio (RER) greater than

Box 2
Workflow to perform an iCPET study

Workflow for an iCPET Study

Initial Referral

- Referral from Pulmonary, Cardiology, Rheumatology, Internal Medicine, and so forth, usually via email, text or through the electronic medical record.

- Decision made whether patient requires an initial clinic visit or iCPET can be performed.

- Computer orders entered which includes right heart catheterization, cardiopulmonary exercise testing, pre-procedural laboratories (basic metabolic panel, complete blood count, coagulopathy panel), and then the patient scheduled by the cath laboratory scheduler

- 1 to 2 prior iCPET study nurse coordinator calls patient, provides an outline of expectations for iCPET study, patients are to wear exercise clothing and sneakers, light breakfast is okay, take all medications, inquires about allergies particularly lidocaine (or other similar anesthetics), or latex (tip of the PA catheter is latex). Inquire about anticoagulants, with recommendations about anticoagulation management.

- We meet weekly on fridays to run the list of referrals. We discuss the patients scheduled on tuesday and/or wednesday. We identify potential issues such as allergies to lidocaine, latex, use of anticoagulants, and whether recent spirometry has been performed (within 6 months of the iCPET study).

- Weekly schedules are sent out by the cath laboratory scheduler by email to those involved in the iCPET program.

Day of iCPET Study

Pre-cath and informed consent

- Patients arrive 1 hours to 2 hours prior to the study to the Same Day Procedural Unit.

- Pre-procedural laboratories collected if not already performed prior to arrival

- Patient is transferred to the Cath Laboratory Holding area where informed consent is performed, ECG leads are placed for the CPET study by exercise physiologist

- Simultaneously the cath lab staff is setting up the RHC equipment and cath lab.

- All of the blood gas syringes are labeled with patient identifying stickers and stage. They are placed on a blue towel on a metal tray and held in the control room until the resting RHC is performed.

Pre-procedure set up

- The patient is transferred to the Cardiac Cath Laboratory and consented to research blood sampling before the procedure.

- The patient is then fitted on the bike, instructions are provided by the exercise physiologist. The patient pedals on the bike to assess for steadiness and ability to perform exercise. If the exercise procedure cannot be performed safely, the patient is having difficulty following directions or the patient appears clinically unstable the procedure will be canceled.

- If the patient requires oxygen during the study, we set up the Douglas bag and identify the percent of oxygen required.

- An exercise effort ramp is determined and adjusted based on the patient's abilities

- The 4th intercostal space (3 fingerbreadths below the axilla, with a relaxed shoulder with hands holding the handlebars as if the patient is exercising) is marked with a medical-grade skin marker. The transducer is leveled to the 4th intercostal space with a laser level fixed to an alligator clamp on an IV pole. The clamp height is measured with a measuring tape and above and below the clamp level is marked with blue painter's tape to facilitate rapid placement when the patient returns to the bicycle.

- The patient is then seated on the first half of the hospital recliner with feet firmly planted on the ground. The transducer is laser leveled to the skin mark at the 4th intercostal space and marked with tape on the IV pole.

- If spirometry needs to be performed it is done prior to the placement of catheters.

- The patient is transferred to the cath laboratory table, raised to the proper height for the procedural physician and leveled with the laser level, height is marked on the IV pole with painter's tape. It is important to not to change the cath laboratory table height once the transducer has been leveled to the patient.

- Ultrasound assessment is performed: radial, ulnar arteries of the non-dominant hand, and the right internal jugular vein images are captured and uploaded to the radiology server. If the radial or ulnar arteries are too small the dominant hand vasculature is then assessed, and the procedure is performed on the best site.

- The patient is prepped and draped and prepared for catheter procedures.

- The transducers are zeroed.

- Call the blood gas lab and notify them that the procedure has started.

Arterial and right heart catheterization procedures

- Arterial line is placed under ultrasound guidance.
- The arterial line is secured with a dressing and not sutured in place.
- Right internal jugular catheterization is performed under ultrasound guidance.
- Hemodynamics are assessed including thermodilution and indirect Fick cardiac outputs.
- Research blood samples are collected during the catheterization from the sheath, right atrium, pulmonary artery, radial artery, and pulmonary artery wedge position at supine rest.
- The right internal jugular cardiac cath is dressed and secured.

Preparation for exercise testing

- The patient is seated at the end of the cath laboratory table and assessed for dizziness.
- The swan is then secured to the patient's right shoulder/back with a large tegaderm.
- The patient is assisted down from the cath laboratory table and takes two steps to the recliner chair and seated as previously instructed. The ECG belt is placed on the patient.
- The transducer is leveled.
- The patient is provided with exercise instructions and the mouthpiece and nose clip is placed. We typically use a mouthpiece, however, if the patient is edentulous or may have trouble keeping the mouthpiece in place we can transition to a mask.
- The blood gas tray is brought into the cath laboratory, and set up with 4 x 4 sponges, labeled syringes to collect peak and post-exercise research blood.
- The PA catheter double gang is prepped for blood gas collection and the rest PA blood gas is connected.
- The patient sits for 5 minutes.
- Call the blood gas lab to notify that the blood gases will be delivered soon.

Performance of iCPET study

- Hemodynamics are collected by the cath laboratory nurse
- Resting RA, RV and PA waveforms are snapped.

- Resting RA, RV and PW waveforms are snapped.
- I hand the arterial blood gas syringe to the cath laboratory tech before each stage to avoid using the wrong stage blood gas.
- Blood from the PA and radial arteries are simultaneously collected and time is noted by the exercise physiologist. I will typically say "pull" to bring blood into the catheters and "draw" to fill the syringe. Time is collected at the time of the "draw". This time is representative of the time of the stage of exercise.
- The patient is then stood up, the exercise bicycle is then slid toward the patient, and the patient is then seated on the bicycle.
- The transducer is leveled and the patient begins exercise.
- Hemodynamics and blood gas are collected at stages of freewheel, 1 to peak exercise in the same order and manner as rest.
- Blood is grouped into 2 sets (4 syringes per set) and run down 4 flights of stairs to be processed in the blood gas lab by respiratory therapy: rest and freewheel, stage 1 and 2, stage 3 and 4, stage 5 and post-exercise.
- Goal for peak exercise is an RER greater than 1.15 or when the patient can no longer keep a pace of 60 RPMs.
- Peak exercise research blood samples are collected immediately after blood gases, and simultaneously from the RA, PA and radial artery.
- The patient performs a 3-min cool down.

Pre-syncope and syncope management plan

- Throughout exercise and particularly post-peak exercise patients are assessed for signs of pre-syncope.
- We follow the patient's systemic pressures from the arterial line, as well as the patient's eye expression. We have noticed that patients who have a blunted stare, cannot focus or maintain attention, or have the "1000-mile stare" are at risk or will have a syncopal episode, even if they continue to pedal and hold onto the handlebars.
- The goal here is to do no harm. If a patient appears pre-syncopal or has a syncopal event the key is to remain calm. The procedural physician must lead the team during the event. Extra staff is called into the room to assist.

- The patient is quickly transitioned from the bicycle to the reclining chair where they are reclined, and their legs are lifted into the air; they are then bolused with IV fluids through the introducer. The patient is assessed during this procedure. All patients will be revived in this manner. Some patients finish the 1L of IV fluids, others can be stopped early.
- If this occurs, we typically are unable to draw post-exercise hemodynamics and physiologic parameters as the mouthpiece has been removed.

Post-exercise

- The patient is seated in the recliner chair in the upright position.
- After 2 minutes of sitting, 5 minutes total post-exercise, we obtain hemodynamics and blood gases, as well as study blood samples.
- Once all of the post-exercise data is collected, I remove the arterial line while the patient is seated, and a TR band is placed; the TE band remains inflated for 20 to 30 minutes and is removed by the heme tech in the cath laboratory holding area.
- The patient is laid supine onto the cath laboratory stretcher the swan is removed and then I remove the introducer and hold pressure for 10 minutes with an occlusive dressing.
- The patient is transferred to the cath laboratory holding area.

Post-procedure data collection

- Blood gas results are manually transposed from the computer to a blood gas work sheet from the post-doctoral research fellow.
- Data is entered into Exper cath laboratory program to calculate the cardiac output values for each stage.
- I work with the exercise physiologist to determine the anaerobic threshold, peak exercise and duration of exercise. The data is exported from the MGC diagnostics Breezesuite program to our homegrown PFT and CPET interpretation program PIMS (pulmonary information management system).
- I overread all of the hemodynamic waveforms and values collected during the study and transpose the values to a hemodynamic worksheet.
- The patients hemodynamic, blood gas and physiologic data are entered into PIMS by the exercise physiologist, finalized and is ready for interpretation.
- I then speak with the patient and family about the procedure, and any preliminary findings.
- I read the iCPET study at a later time. Referring physicians are notified about the study results. Patients are either notified electronically or by phone regarding the results and a plan is enacted.

This is an example of our specific workflow at the University of Pittsburgh at our Shadyside site.

or equal to 1.15 but depending on the effort we accept an RER greater than 1.10, particularly in those patients experiencing a decrement in the rotations per minute approaching peak exercise.

We obtain hemodynamic, blood gas, and CPET values at rest after 5 minutes of seated, undisturbed breathing to ensure that we have true resting measures. Patients are encouraged not to talk throughout the study as it will disturb our hemodynamic measurements. They are shown hand signs to convey symptoms of dizziness, chest pain, and so forth. The zero reference level in the upright position is the 4th intercostal space.[6] Our hemodynamic measurements are recorded with Xper Cardio Physiomonitoring System (Philips, Melbourne, FL, USA) in the rest seated, unloaded pedaling, and every 2 minutes during exercise through peak (which is approximately 4–5 stages depending on the patient's abilities). Hemodynamic measurements are averaged over 3 to 4 respiratory cycles.[34] We calculate direct Fick CO as $CO = VO_2/(SaO_2-SmvO_2)*1.36*Hb_a*10$, at rest seated and at each aforementioned stage of exercise. In the Fick equation, SaO_2 is arterial saturation, $SmvO_2$ is mixed venous saturation, and Hb_a is arterial hemoglobin in g/dL. Blood gas samples are collected from the radial artery line and distal port of the PA catheter at each stage. We collect the modified Borg rating of perceived exertion at each stage of the study.

What Will Your Role Be?

To succeed in this role, you will need to undertake the following tasks.

1. Provide Informed Consent: Ensure patients understand the procedure.
2. Consent for Research Studies: Obtain consent for research participation.
3. Place Arterial Line and PA Catheter: Troubleshoot equipment and transducers while maintaining sterility.

4. Perform Right Heart Catheterization: Conduct the catheterization procedure.
5. Run the Room During Exercise Study: Lead operations during the exercise study.
6. Know All Roles and Equipment: Understand all jobs in the room, tubing connections, and CPET machine functions, and troubleshoot any issues. Lead from the ground floor.
7. Ensure Proper Data Collection: Verify that all data are accurately collected.
8. Interpret the Studies: Analyze and interpret the study results.
9. Meet with the iCPET Team Regularly: Ensure the program functions smoothly, address concerns, and manage patient referrals and scheduling.

Here are 7 essential and binding rules to remember when performing iCPET studies to ensure the success of the program.

1. There are no do-overs. Think of the iCPET study as an unstoppable train. Once the mouthpiece is in and the patient has started exercising, the study cannot be interrupted. All processes and workflow should be developed to preclude any interruptions during the study.
2. Make sure the study is interpretable. The patient has been referred to you to identify the etiology of their dyspnea or exercise intolerance. It is up to you to ensure that the test can provide an answer. The best way to do this is to set the patient's expectations before the study, preferably at the time of informed consent, and reinforce the goals during the study. For example, we explain that the patient should not stop pedaling during the study, attempt to talk while the mouthpiece is in place, remove it prematurely, or perform a submaximal study.
3. Set expectations. At the time of consent, it is crucial to review the study process in detail, covering catheter(s) placement, the exercise study, and recovery. Discuss potential diagnoses, considering the patient's medical history, and highlight that the study might show normal physiology or deconditioning. Note that normal peak oxygen consumption (VO_2) can coexist with other abnormalities, especially in patients with Long-COVID,[9] or chronic thromboembolic disease,[35] (where a normal peak VO_2 is achieved, but abnormally increased dead space is present). Inform patients that deconditioning is curable, unlike many other physiologic issues. Having this discussion to set up expectations before the exercise study is essential for patient understanding.
4. Do no harm. Ensuring patient safety is paramount. As an outpatient procedure, patients expect to go home afterward. Our goal is to place the arterial line and PA catheter with a single needle stick, avoiding vascular injury. Careful assessment of hand perfusion during and after the study is essential. Additionally, if a patient does not appear stable or able to perform the exercise study safely, the procedure should be canceled or rescheduled.
5. Create a rapport with the patient. Most, if not all, patients will be anxious before and during the study. After the study, you will notice the heart rate, blood pressure, and minute ventilation have improved. For the most part, we have been able to keep patients comfortable during their study. In addition, we make jokes and keep the mood in the room light while still maintaining a professional atmosphere. We establish expectations before the procedure, we address all concerns as they arise. It is a difficult line to walk, particularly since you will need to perform all procedures meticulously, oversee the staff, care for the patient, and provide oversight for the study.
6. Interpret the study in detail. Review the study. Take your time interpreting the data. Make sure that the physiology makes sense, and make sure that you have considered all the possible diagnoses based on your findings. Then, once a differential or a definitive diagnosis has been reported, leave recommendations for further studies that may confirm your conclusions (ie, a VQ scan to identify chronic pulmonary embolism, in a patient with dyspnea and increased dead space during exercise).
7. Get help when you need it. For those who already know how to interpret a non-invasive CPET, interpretation of the 9-panel plot generated by an iCPET will not pose a challenge. Similarly, providers who are well-versed in the assessment of a resting right heart catheterization or a more basic supine or semi-recumbent exercise right heart catheterization will quickly master the nuances of interpreting the hemodynamics generated during an iCPET. However, few individuals are comfortable interpreting both the gas exchange and hemodynamic patterns produced by an iCPET when they first start a program. Do not be intimidated by the large amount of initially unfamiliar data generated by the study. Instead, consider instituting a team-based approach to iCPET interpretation. Giving each member of the team time to examine the data independently and then convening a group interpretation session to share thoughts facilitates a cross-pollination of ideas and approaches that will benefit everyone's maturation into iCPET experts.

HOW IS THE ROOM GOING TO BE SET UP?

The set-up of the room may depend on where the iCPET studies are performed. **Fig. 1** shows pictures of a typical iCPET study. The key to performing the study in a single room is the proximity of the metabolic cart to the cath laboratory table and a reclining chair (which is where the patient sits for the resting stage assessment). This ensures that the patient will not need to travel far when moving from one portion of the study to another. Before performing an iCPET study, set up your iCPET work triangle.

WHO IS GOING TO PROCESS THE BLOOD GASES?

There will be a lot of blood gases to process. We gather hemodynamic and blood samples after each 2-min exercise stage, and patients usually perform 4 or 5 stages of exercise. In addition, we add rest, freewheel (a warmup stage during which the motor of the ergometer drives the pedals), and post-exercise stages. This results in up to 16 blood gases being drawn, and processing of the samples can be time-consuming.

There are 2 options for blood gas processing. The first is to deliver batched samples to the laboratory over the course of the exercise study. We utilize the approach, which involves drawing an arterial blood gas and venous blood gas during each stage, and sending the samples to the laboratory after every 2 stages (4 samples per batch) utilizing a "runner." This requires a staff member to run the samples, and troubleshoot any issues as they arise in real time, during an exercise study. For each sample we order a blood gas (pH, $Paco_2$, Pao_2), oximetry (O_2 saturation, hemoglobin), electrolytes (bicarbonate, base excess/deficit), and metabolites (lactate).

Blood gas analysis can be performed in a central laboratory, a separate blood gas laboratory (our situation), or by a blood gas machine in the cath laboratory. In each case, a formalized quality control program must be in place; this is an important factor to consider if an iCPET program is considering the purchase of a blood gas machine specifically for that program. We do not utilize the tube system for sending blood gas samples to the laboratory out of concern that it could result in sample loss or a delay in processing. Programs should

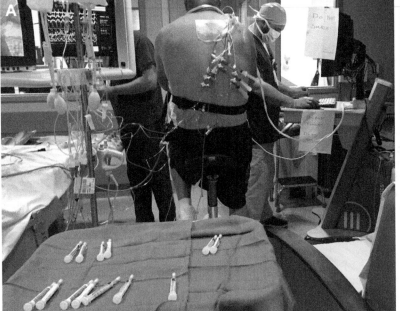
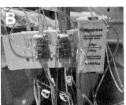
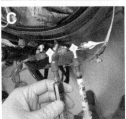
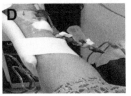

Fig. 1. (*A*) Set-up of the invasive cardiopulmonary exercise testing study in the cardiac cath laboratory. The patient is seated on the exercise bicycle in the center of the picture. To the left of the patient is the cath laboratory table, monitor, the IV pole with transducers, and the cath laboratory nurse collecting blood from the arterial line. To the right of the patient is one of our exercise physiologists working with the MGC diagnostics metabolic cart. On the right closer to the foreground is the reclining chair where the patient sits for rest seated and post-exercise measurements. (*B*) Transducers on an alligator clip attached to an IV pole for a VIP swan with RA, RV, PA and arterial line transducers from left to right. (*C*) A double gang set up for the pulmonary artery channel. This allows for the saline and blood from the catheter to be withdrawn into a 10 mL syringe so only blood can be collected in the blood gas syringe. (*D*) Possible set-up for the radial artery catheter which allows blood pressures to be transduced, and samples can be retrieved. Alternatively, a vamp system can be set up to collect blood gas samples.

consider collecting duplicate samples at resting and peak exercise to ensure accurate measurements for these critical stages.

REFERRALS AND ORDERS

What will your referral process be like? How will other physicians know that you have a program? Will you advertise? Will you give Grand Rounds? Keep track of your referral sources. Eventually, after notifying potential referral sources that you have established a program, you will have patients sent to you. Make sure you cultivate relationships with referring providers; make sure that they can get in touch with you and consider providing your email or cell phone number to referring physicians. We track the referrals on a shared excel spreadsheet, which helps us manage our referral network.

Make sure that you establish a formalized process for ordering a iCPET. Our institution utilizes Epic (Verona, Wisconsin, USA) for outpatient notes and orders. You should meet with the electronic medical record (EMR) programmers to create an order set that makes it easy for referring providers to order a study.

SO, YOU WANT TO DO RESEARCH?

Accumulating enough iCPET studies to answer research questions and publish data takes years. Our volume remained consistent at 60 to 70 studies per year. The coronavirus disease 2019 (COVID-19) pandemic disrupted our progress but provided enough post-acute sequelae of COVID-19 (PASC) patients to publish our findings,[25] with our first iCPET manuscript published 7 years after starting the program. Unless your referrals are sourced from a single population, such as heart failure or chronic pulmonary embolism, they will likely be heterogeneous, making it challenging to publish due to small cohort sizes. Additionally, obtaining a control group with normal physiology can be difficult.

Be persistent in applying for funding. Whether it is federal, private or clinical trial funding, the research engine of the program will allow for growth and ongoing productivity. I have had success receiving generous funding from the Shadyside Foundation, which has been a tremendous help in covering portions of the salaries of my staff and sustaining the iCPET program.

SUMMARY

I am over 6 years into establishing the iCPET program at UPMC. I feel that we are only now starting to gain some programmatic momentum, particularly with our research endeavors.

The establishment of an iCPET program demands meticulous planning, collaboration among diverse stakeholders, and a commitment to patient safety. While the benefits of diagnostic precision and personalized treatment strategies are substantial, the inherent challenges in establishing and maintaining a program necessitate the early development of comprehensive, thoughtful clinical and business plans. With a well-structured approach and a dedicated team, an iCPET program can become a cornerstone in advancing cardiovascular and pulmonary medicine. I have found joy in establishing the program, working with wonderful people, and performing and interpreting physiology-based testing.

WAS IT WORTH IT?

No doubt: yes.

CLINICS CARE POINTS

- Patient Selection and Referral: Ensure careful selection and referral of patients to the iCPET program, prioritizing those with unexplained exercise intolerance and dyspnea where previous diagnostic tests have been inconclusive.

- Risk Management: Be vigilant about the invasive nature of iCPET; understand the inherent risks and ensure all procedural safeguards are in place to manage potential complications.

- Training and Competency: Maintain a high standard of training and competency among staff conducting iCPET to ensure accurate data collection and interpretation, which are critical for effective patient diagnosis and management.

- Follow-Up and Documentation: Implement rigorous follow-up procedures and thorough documentation practices to monitor patient outcomes and program efficacy.

DISCLOSURE

Dr M.G. Risbano receives grant support for the iCPET program from Shadyside Hospital Foundation.

REFERENCES

1. Wallace WD, Nouraie M, Chan SY, et al. Treatment of exercise pulmonary hypertension improves

pulmonary vascular distensibility. Pulm Circ 2018; 8(3). 2045894018787381.

2. Zhao J, Florentin J, Tai YY, et al. Long range endocrine delivery of circulating mir-210 to endothelium promotes pulmonary hypertension. Circ Res 2020; 127(5):677–92.

3. Zou RH, Wallace WD, Nouraie SM, et al. Lower DLco % identifies exercise pulmonary hypertension in patients with parenchymal lung disease referred for dyspnea. Pulm Circ 2020;10(1). 2045894019891912.

4. Huang W, Resch S, Oliveira RK, et al. Invasive cardiopulmonary exercise testing in the evaluation of unexplained dyspnea: Insights from a multidisciplinary dyspnea center. Eur J Prev Cardiol 2017; 24(11):1190–9.

5. Berry NC, Manyoo A, Oldham WM, et al. Protocol for exercise hemodynamic assessment: performing an invasive cardiopulmonary exercise test in clinical practice. Pulm Circ 2015;5(4):610–8.

6. Maron BA, Cockrill BA, Waxman AB, et al. The invasive cardiopulmonary exercise test. Circulation 2013;127(10):1157–64.

7. Lewis GD, Bossone E, Naeije R, et al. Pulmonary vascular hemodynamic response to exercise in cardiopulmonary diseases. Circulation 2013;128(13): 1470–9.

8. Kovacs G, Herve P, Barbera JA, et al. An official European Respiratory Society statement: pulmonary haemodynamics during exercise. Eur Respir J 2017;50(5).

9. Risbano MG, Kliment CR, Dunlap DG, et al. Postacute Sequelae of SARS-CoV-2 Infection Patients Have Metabolic Reprogramming and Reduced Mitochondrial Function at Peak Exercise. Am J Respir Crit Care Med 2023;207.

10. Faria-Urbina M, Oliveira RKF, Segrera SA, et al. Impaired systemic oxygen extraction in treated exercise pulmonary hypertension: a new engine in an old car? Pulm Circ 2018;8(1). 2045893218755325.

11. Naeije R, Vanderpool R, Dhakal BP, et al. Exercise-induced pulmonary hypertension: physiological basis and methodological concerns. Am J Respir Crit Care Med 2013;187(6):576–83.

12. Segrera SA, Lawler L, Opotowsky AR, et al. Open label study of ambrisentan in patients with exercise pulmonary hypertension. Pulm Circ 2017;7(2):531–8.

13. Tolle JJ, Waxman AB, Van Horn TL, et al. Exercise-induced pulmonary arterial hypertension. Circulation 2008;118(21):2183–9.

14. Ho JE, Zern EK, Lau ES, et al. Exercise pulmonary hypertension predicts clinical outcomes in patients with dyspnea on effort. J Am Coll Cardiol 2020; 75(1):17–26.

15. Naeije R, Boerrigter BG. Pulmonary hypertension at exercise in COPD: does it matter? Eur Respir J 2013; 41(5):1002–4.

16. Oliveira RK, Agarwal M, Tracy JA, et al. Age-related upper limits of normal for maximum upright exercise

17. Herve P, Lau EM, Sitbon O, et al. Criteria for diagnosis of exercise pulmonary hypertension. Eur Respir J 2015;46(3):728–37.

18. Morris TA, Fernandes TM, Channick RN. Evaluation of dyspnea and exercise intolerance after acute pulmonary embolism. Chest 2023;163(4): 933–41.

19. Borlaug BA, Nishimura RA, Sorajja P, et al. Exercise hemodynamics enhance diagnosis of early heart failure with preserved ejection fraction. Circ Heart Fail 2010;3(5):588–95.

20. Gorter TM, Obokata M, Reddy YNV, et al. Exercise unmasks distinct pathophysiologic features in heart failure with preserved ejection fraction and pulmonary vascular disease. Eur Heart J 2018;39(30): 2825–35.

21. Malhotra R, Dhakal BP, Eisman AS, et al. Pulmonary vascular distensibility predicts pulmonary hypertension severity, exercise capacity, and survival in heart failure. Circ Heart Fail 2016;9(6).

22. Lewis GD, Murphy RM, Shah RV, et al. Pulmonary vascular response patterns during exercise in left ventricular systolic dysfunction predict exercise capacity and outcomes. Circ Heart Fail 2011;4(3): 276–85.

23. Hilde JM, Skjorten I, Hansteen V, et al. Haemodynamic responses to exercise in patients with COPD. Eur Respir J 2013;41(5):1031–41.

24. Tolle J, Waxman A, Systrom D. Impaired systemic oxygen extraction at maximum exercise in pulmonary hypertension. Med Sci Sports Exerc 2008; 40(1):3–8.

25. Risbano MG, Kliment CR, Dunlap DG, et al. Invasive cardiopulmonary exercise testing identifies distinct physiologic endotypes in post-acute sequelae of SARS-CoV-2 infection. Chest Pulmonary 2023;1(3): 1–16.

26. Oldham WM, Lewis GD, Opotowsky AR, et al. Unexplained exertional dyspnea caused by low ventricular filling pressures: results from clinical invasive cardiopulmonary exercise testing. Pulm Circ 2016; 6(1):55–62.

27. Simonneau G, Montani D, Celermajer DS, et al. Haemodynamic definitions and updated clinical classification of pulmonary hypertension. Eur Respir J 2019;53(1).

28. Campedelli L, Nouraie SM, Risbano MG. Non-arterial line cardiac output calculation misclassifies exercise pulmonary hypertension and increases risk of data loss particularly in black, Scleroderma, and Raynaud's patients during invasive exercise testing. Eur Respir J 2024;64. https://doi.org/10.1183/ 13993003.02232-2023.

29. Naeije R, Chesler N. Pulmonary circulation at exercise. Compr Physiol 2012;2(1):711–41.

30. Kirupaharan P, Lane J, Melillo C, et al. Impact of body position on hemodynamic measurements during exercise: A tale of two bikes. Pulm Circ 2024; 14(1):e12334.

31. Walsh-Riddle M, Blumenthal JA. Cardiovascular responses during upright and semi-recumbent cycle ergometry testing. Med Sci Sports Exerc 1989; 21(5):581–5.

32. Wehrle A, Waibel S, Gollhofer A, et al. Power output and efficiency during supine, recumbent, and upright cycle ergometry. Front Sports Act Living 2021;3:667564.

33. Kovacs G, Avian A, Olschewski A, et al. Zero reference level for right heart catheterisation. Eur Respir J 2013;42(6):1586–94.

34. Boerrigter BG, Waxman AB, Westerhof N, et al. Measuring central pulmonary pressures during exercise in COPD: how to cope with respiratory effects. Eur Respir J 2014;43(5):1316–25.

35. Fernandes TM, Alotaibi M, Strozza DM, et al. Dyspnea postpulmonary embolism from physiological dead space proportion and stroke volume defects during exercise. Chest 2020;157(4):936–44.

Cardiopulmonary Exercise Testing in Research

Alexandria Miller, MD[a], Rebecca R. Vanderpool, PhD[b],*

KEYWORDS

- Exercise hemodynamics ● Heart failure with preserved ejection fraction ● Pulmonary hypertension

KEY POINTS

- Noninvasive and invasive cardiopulmonary exercise testing is important for the diagnosis and phenotyping of exercise intolerance in complex diseases like heart failure and pulmonary hypertension.
- Current research efforts focus on quantifying underlying changes in the cardiopulmonary pathophysiology of exercise intolerance to more precisely phenotype patients to personalize medicine.
- Cardiopulmonary exercise testing generates a wealth of information, but additional validation and noninvasive measures are needed to bring these metrics into standard clinical practice.

INTRODUCTION

Cardiopulmonary exercise testing (CPET) is a form of stress testing that is commonly used in the evaluation of unexplained dyspnea, as well as for prognostication in patients with cardiopulmonary disease processes. Both noninvasive and invasive CPET assess functional capacity, ventilatory efficiency, gas exchange, and cardiac function; invasive CPET provides additional diagnostic utility through placement of radial artery and pulmonary artery catheters to assess hemodynamics during graded exercise. Pulmonary hypertension is highly prevalent in heart failure populations, with a smaller subset developing pulmonary vascular disease (PVD) that portends a worse prognosis.[1] In recent years, the applicability of CPET to aid in the diagnosis of challenging disease processes has grown, with continued researching focusing on novel hemodynamic parameters to further characterize various disease states and influence therapeutics and prognosis.

RESEARCH APPLICATIONS OF EXERCISE TESTING: ELUCIDATING PATHOPHYSIOLOGY

CPET has been well established as a tool for the evaluation of patients with unexplained dyspnea and heart failure with reduced ejection fraction.[2] Noninvasive CPET has the ability to help differentiate limitations due to deconditioning or cardiac or pulmonary etiologies. Typical noninvasive CPET parameters include peak oxygen consumption (V_{O_2}), carbon dioxide production (VCO_2), exercise ventilation (VE), and end tidal oxygen (O_2) and carbon dioxide (CO_2). Additional derived parameters include the tidal volume (VE/RR), ventilatory equivalent for oxygen (VE/V_{O_2}) and carbon dioxide (VE/VCO_2), and O_2 pulse (V_{O_2}/heart rate) (**Fig. 1**). The addition of invasive hemodynamics to CPET allows for further evaluation of hemodynamics, as well as oxygen extraction and utilization with exercise.[3]

In recent years, these tests have significantly expanded our ability to diagnose heart failure with

a Department of Cardiology, The Ohio State University Wexner Medical Center, Davis Heart and Lung Research Institute, Suite 200, 473 West 12th Avenue, Columbus, OH 43210, USA; b Division of Cardiovascular Medicine, The Ohio State University Wexner Medical Center, Davis Heart and Lung Research Institute, Suite 611b 473 West 12th Avenue, Columbus, OH 43210, USA
* Corresponding author.
E-mail address: Rebecca.Vanderpool@osumc.edu

Heart Failure Clin 21 (2025) 111–117
https://doi.org/10.1016/j.hfc.2024.09.002
1551-7136/25/© 2024 Elsevier Inc. All rights are reserved, including those for text and data mining, AI training, and similar technologies.

Cardiopulmonary Exercise Test Parameters

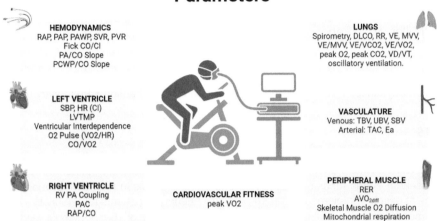

Fig. 1. Functional parameters that can be obtained on noninvasive or invasive cardiopulmonary exercise testing. The identified functional parameters associate with hemodynamics, left and right ventricular function, pulmonary function, and changes in the systemic system that assist with the diagnosis and phenotyping of complex syndromes like exercise intolerance, heart failure, and pulmonary hypertension. AVO_{2diff}, arterial to venous oxygen saturation difference; CI, cardiac index; CI, chronotropic incompetence; CO, cardiac output; DLCO, diffusion capacity of lungs for carbon monoxide; Ea, arterial elastance; HR, heart rate; MVV, maximal voluntary ventilation; PA, pulmonary artery; PAC, pulmonary arterial compliance; PAP, pulmonary arterial pressure; PAWP, pulmonary Artery wedge pressure; PVR, pulmonary vascular resistance; RAP, right atrial pressure; RER, respiratory exchange ratio; RR, respiratory rate; RV, Right ventricle; SBP, systolic blood pressure; SBV, stress blood volume; SVR, systemic vascular resistance; TAC, total arterial compliance; TBV, total blood volume; UBV, unstressed blood volume; VD/VT, dead space ventilation ratio; VE, ventilatory equivalent; VE/VCO_2, ventilatory equivalent for carbon monoxide; VE/Vo_2, ventilatory equivalent for oxygen. (Created in BioRender. Vanderpool, R. (2024) BioRender.com/a96p436.)

preserved ejection fraction (HFpEF) and exercise pulmonary hypertension (PH). Proposed diagnostic algorithms for HFpEF including the H2FPEF score and HFA-PEFF algorithms include diastolic stress echocardiography and exercise right heart catheterization for those with intermediate risk scores.[4,5] CPET, particularly invasive CPET, is not emphasized in the current diagnostic algorithms despite increasing research of its utility.[4,5] The growing use of invasive CPET in recent years has led to substantial research regarding this form of exercise testing to better understand the pathophysiologic disturbances in patients with unexplained dyspnea. While the hemodynamics definition of HFpEF and exercise-induced PH has been refined over recent years, particularly with serial measurements to define pulmonary artery wedge pressure to cardiac output (PAWP/CO) and mean PA pressure to cardiac output (mPAP/CO) slopes,[5–7] several invasive CPET parameters represent areas of research interest aimed at better defining the pathophysiology of these disease states.

Several novel markers that are being researched to better define the pathophysiology and subgroups of HFpEF patients include arterial stiffness,

venous compliance, and impairments in the oxygen extraction pathway. Arterial stiffness is a load-independent marker that is measured invasively as total arterial compliance (TAC) and arterial elastance (Ea). Arterial stiffness has been known to increase with hypertensive disease and also normal aging that are both common comorbidities in patients with HFpEF.[8] Reddy and colleagues subsequently studied the differences in arterial stiffness and compliance between HFpEF and hypertensive controls with invasive CPET. This study showed that while these 2 groups of patients had similar mean arterial pressures and arterial stiffness at rest, with exercise patients with HFpEF had less reduction in systemic vascular resistance, lower TAC, and higher Ea that correlated with increased PAWP and reduced cardiac output. They advocated that this finding could suggest a therapeutic target for patients with HFpEF.[8]

Venous capacitance is important for modulation of blood volume at rest and during exercise with total body volume made up of unstressed blood volume and stress blood volume that can be mobilized with exercise and sympathetic activation. Sorimachi and colleagues performed invasive cardiopulmonary exercise testing (iCPET) and echocardiography to evaluate changes in venous capacitance in patients with HFpEF versus noncardiac dyspnea. Patients with HFpEF were found to have decreased venous capacitance and increased stress blood volumes compared to patients with noncardiac dyspnea. Despite this increase in stress blood volume, patients with HFpEF also showed decreased augmentation of cardiac output. These findings were more significant with increased body mass index.[9] Similarly, in a study looking at the invasive exercise hemodynamics between patients with PAH, PH-HFpEF, and controls, they found that patients with PH-HFpEF had evidence of increase right atrial (RA)/CO slope, RA pressure, and increased stress blood volume compared to both PAH and control patients.[10] These studies again help better define distinct pathophysiologic methods in the heterogenous population of patients with HFpEF.

Exercise studies have also been used to explore the role of oxygen extraction in pathophysiologic adaptations in HFpEF. An iCPET-based study by Dhakal and colleagues[11] showed that, in comparison to patients with HFrEF, the biggest determinants of decrease Vo_2 in patients with HFpEF were related to lower peripheral oxygen extraction and peak heart rate. Houstis and colleagues took this analysis a step further and found that patients with HFpEF had defects in several steps along the pathway of oxygen utilization and extraction with exercise. They also found that there was significant heterogeneity to the defects present in each patient, as well as individualized differences in how improvement in these defects improved Vo_2.[12] These findings highlight the ways in which iCPET is being used to both identify pathophysiologic mechanisms in patients with HFpEF and identify possible therapeutic targets.

An additional area of research interest is the use of invasive CPET to better understand the contribution of PVD in patients with HFpEF. HFpEF is associated with PH in up to 80% of patients and can have associated PVD as defined by pulmonary vascular resistance (PVR) greater than 2 to 3 WU at rest or PVR greater than 1.74 WU with exercise, which portends a worse prognosis.[1] Several parameters have been explored in an effort to better understand the pathophysiology of these patients. Patients with HFpEF and PVD have been found to have increased right ventricular to pulmonary arterial (RV-PA) uncoupling and tricuspid regurgitation, increased right atrial pressure with exercise, decreased pulmonary artery compliance, increased dead space ventilation (VD/VT), decreased left ventricular transmural pressure,

and increased interventricular dependence with exercise, compared to those with isolated post-capillary PH. The combination of these findings leads to a decreased ability to augment stroke volume with exercise and also reduced exercise capacity.[1,13,14] Being able to identify this subgroup of patients with invasive measures is important when considering therapeutic options and defining prognosis.

Given the vast information that can be obtained from noninvasive and particularly invasive CPET, Guazzi and colleagues advocated for the incorporation of CPET into the HFA-PEFF algorithm in a recent clinical consensus statement of the Heart Failure Association and European Association of Preventative Cardiology of the European Society of Cardiology. They recommended use at the pre-assessment point to evaluate for alternative diagnoses if HFpEF is ruled out, as well as in the final step of the algorithm to characterize the pathophysiologic defects in patients with HFpEF, guide therapeutics, and assist with prognosis.[15]

RESEARCH APPLICATIONS OF EXERCISE TESTING: IDENTIFCATION OF NOVEL ENDOPHENOTYPES

Complex diseases including heart failure and PH have heterogeneity in their clinical presentation and underlying cardiopulmonary physiology (**Fig. 2**). Current assessments that focus on PVR and pressure-flow relationships including mPAP/CO and PAWP/CO slope only characterize the steady component of pulmonary arterial afterload.[16] Pulmonary vascular impedance is a more complete description of pulmonary arterial afterload that incorporates steady (input impedance) and pulsatile (characteristic impedance) components of the afterload. Under normal conditions, the pulmonary vasculature is a highly compliant system that accommodates high flow at low pressure.[17] Consequences of pulmonary vascular remodeling include a reduction of the radius of vessels as well as a decrease in pulmonary vascular compliance. Pulmonary vascular compliance can be broken down into measures of proximal distensibility (beta), global compliance (stroke volume/pulse pressure), and distal vessel distensibility (alpha distensibility).[18–20] Pressure–volume loops are the gold standard for quantifying RV adaptation to alterations in arterial afterload with measures of end-systolic elastance (Ees: RV contractility), Ea, RV-PA coupling ratio (Ees/Ea), RV stroke work, and RV power.[21] The more complex descriptions of the pulmonary circulation including the pulsatile load, RV pressure–volume loops, and distensibility α are mainly used in

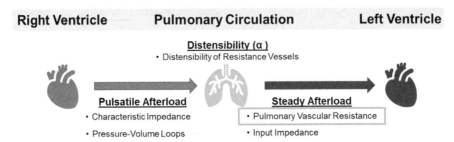

Fig. 2. Research methods to assess pulmonary vascular afterload and right ventricular function. Current clinical methods and guidelines use pulmonary vascular resistance (outlined in *green*) to quantify pulmonary arterial afterload. Additional physiologic information including pulsatile afterload, RV function from pressure–volume loops, and distal vascular distensibility measurements can be used to more precisely phenotype patients.

translational research studies to better phenotype patients. Before these complex metrics can be utilized in standard clinical practices, methods and clinically meaningful values need to be standardized across centers.[22,23]

PVD in the setting of heart failure or PH is associated with increased hospitalization and mortality.[24] Resting hemodynamic metrics of PVD include PVR, transpulmonary gradient and the diastolic pulmonary gradient are hemodynamic markers that associate with pulmonary vascular remodeling but they only describe changes in the steady component of arterial afterload.

Pressure-flow measurements at multiple exercise stages during an iCPET can be used to quantify distal vascular remodeling with the quantification of the pulmonary vascular distensibility.[17] Alpha distensibility coefficient is determined from a nonlinear fit to multipoint pressure-flow plots. Studies have demonstrated that patients with heart failure (0.8%–0.9%) and PAH (0.4%) have decreased distensibility compared to patients with normal pulmonary pressure (α: 1%–2%).[25]

Distensibility (α) has been used for the early detection of PVD,[17,26,27] as well as differentiating PAH from left-sided heart failure.[25] It also associates with outcomes in patients with borderline PH and heart failure ejection fraction[25,28] and was an independent predictor of peak RV-PA coupling in patients with PAH, exercise PH, and heart failure preserved ejection fraction.[29] Despite being clinically relevant, distensibility (α) is not widely calculated but a recent Web-based analysis tool has been developed to standardize calculations and methods for translation distensibility (α) to more clinical settings.[30] While distensibility (α) is modifiable by vasodilatory therapy in exercise PH[27] and heart failure patients,[25] there were no significant changes in patients with established PH.[30]

Multimodal approaches can also be used to quantify the right ventricular reserve with conductance catheter RV pressure–volume loop assessment during exercise testing.[21,31] In a coupled state, the right ventricle initially adapts to increased afterload with an increase in contractility followed by changes in volume.[32] Conductance catheter RV pressure–volume loops demonstrate different modes and degree of RV reserve in patients with and without heart failure or PH (**Fig. 3**). Participants with normal pressure have minimal changes in pressure with a slight shift to the left. In PH-HFpEF, RV pressure is already increased at the initial exercise stage with a volume shit to the right. Within pulmonary arterial hypertension, right ventricles in patients with idiopathic PAH (IPAH) and systemic sclerosis-associated pulmonary arterial hypertension (SSc-PAH) respond in different ways. Patients with IPAH have a slight increase in pressure with a slight shift to the left in volume. In contrast, SSc-PAH has a progressive increase in pressure with a shit of volumes to the right or higher volumes.[21] Quantification of these changes in RV function in combination with changes in the pulmonary circulation will allow clinicians to highly phenotype their patients to better understand the pathophysiological of cardiac-related exercise intolerance to better personalize therapeutic strategies.[33]

Currently, there is no standard protocol for noninvasive and invasive CPET testing. These studies are performed under slightly different conditions at each center, making it difficult to include exercise testing in clinical guidelines or to identify clinically meaningful cut-offs. The Pulmonary Vascular Disease Phenomics (PVDOMICS) study is the first consortium effort to standardize CPET protocols across centers in a large cohort of participants with a variety of mixed PVD phenotypes including disease comparators.[34] In their published protocol,[34] the investigators highlight the importance of (1) standardizing which pressure tracings were captured including the RA, the RV, and the pulmonary wedge position and (2) zero referencing the pressure transducers at the mid-

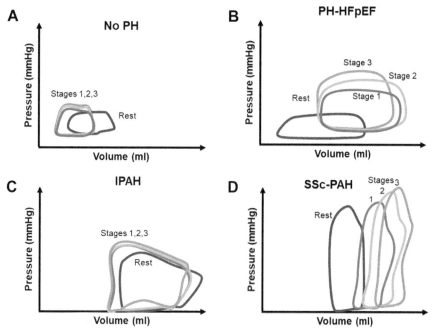

Fig. 3. Right ventricular pressure–volume function during exercise testing. Representative changes in conductance catheter measurements of right ventricular pressure–volume loops demonstrate different modes of adaptation to exercise and afterload in patients with (A) no pulmonary hypertension,[21] (B) pulmonary hypertension in the setting of heart failure preserved ejection fraction (PH-HFpEF),[31] (C) idiopathic pulmonary arterial hypertension (IPAH),[21] and (D) systemic sclerosis-associated pulmonary arterial hypertension (SSc-PAH).[21]

thoracic level as the best approximation of the left atrium with releveling when the participant is in the upright position.[35] Proper placement of the radial catheter for arterial oxygen saturations is important for accurate determination of Fick cardiac output during exercise so as to avoid misclassification of exercise PH.[36] An example of an iCPET protocol, as well as advice on how to perform the study, is included in the article, "The Invasive Cardiopulmonary Exercise Test: A Practical Guide" in this issue of heart failure clinics. Additional efforts to standardize and disseminate a universal iCPET protocol, identify advanced hemodynamic and gas exchange metrics that should be collected during every exercise study, and establish a shared exercise study registry are needed to further both research and clinical use of iCPET.

FUTURE DIRECTIONS

Over the last several years, there has been significant growth in research applications of exercise testing. These efforts have contributed to our ability to diagnose, phenotype, and design therapeutic interventions for patients with unexplained dyspnea and, in particular, those with HFpEF and exercise PH. Despite this advancement, iCPET

remains underutilized due to its complexity, lack of a standardized protocol, and lack of availability outside of tertiary care centers. These issues emphasize the need for noninvasive testing that can provide similar information. Exercise stress echocardiography and the noninvasive CPET are also helpful in the evaluation of this patient population with unexplained dyspnea.[37] Exercise stress echocardiography is a more widely available modality that has the benefit of also being able to rule out alternative etiologies of dyspnea such as coronary artery or valvular disease. Exercise lung ultrasonography has also shown promise in helping to diagnose HFpEF, as the presence of B lines is suggestive of exercise-induced elevation in filling pressures.[37,38] Pugliese and colleagues[39] have used exercise stress echocardiography with simultaneous CPET to show that parameters including left ventricular systolic annulus tissue velocity, right ventricular to PA coupling, and low left atrial reservoir strain/E/e ratio are predictive of low peak V_{O_2}.

Exercise cardiac MR (CMR) imaging is helpful in diagnosing HFpEF, as well as ruling out alternative etiologies for dyspnea including coronary artery and infiltrative cardiomyopathies. The HFpEF Stress trial was a small study by Backhaus and colleagues in 34 patients with HFpEF and found that real-time CMR exercise left atrial long-axis strain as an independent predictor of HFpEF. While this study was limited given its small size and multiple exclusion criteria that included comorbidities frequently seen in patients with HFpEF, it suggests the possibility of exercise real-time CMR in the future to aid in the noninvasive diagnosis of HFpEF.[40]

SUMMARY

CPET, and iCPET in particular, is an evolving area of research in heart failure and exercise PH. While the area has evolved significantly in recent years, additional research efforts aimed at identifying novel parameters useful in diagnosing, phenotyping, and determining prognosis are needed. Deeper phenotyping of patients with heart failure or PH is of critical importance, given the significant heterogeneity of this patient population, and the need to better match patients with appropriate clinical trials.

CLINICS CARE POINTS

- Unexplained dyspnea is a common clinical complaint with multiple possible etiologies. CPET provides data to help refine the differential diagnosis by providing not only additional diagnostic data, but also data useful in the characterization of the underlying pathophysiologic mechanisms that could inform therapeutics and prognosis.

- CPET, and in particular invasive CPET, has not yet been standardized, leading to variations in data obtained and interpretation of results.

- Invasive CPET is not widely available, which limits the current utility of the test for diagnosis of unexplained dyspnea in the general population.

DISCLOSURE

The authors have no disclosures.

REFERENCES

1. Caravita S, Baratto C, Filippo A, et al. Shedding light on latent pulmonary vascular disease in heart failure with preserved ejection fraction. JACC Heart Fail 2023;11:1427–38.
2. Ozemek C, Hardwick J, Bonikowske A, et al. How to interpret a cardiorespiratory fitness assessment – key measures that provide the best picture of health, disease status and prognosis. Prog Cardiovasc Dis 2024;83:23–8.
3. Huang W, Resch S, Oliveira RK, et al. Invasive cardiopulmonary exercise testing in the evaluation of unexplained dyspnea: insights from a multidisciplinary dyspnea center. Eur J Prev Cardiol 2017; 24:1190–9.
4. Reddy YNV, Carter RE, Obokata M, et al. A simple, evidence-based approach to help guide diagnosis of heart failure with preserved ejection fraction. Circulation 2018;138:861–70.
5. Pieske B, Tschöpe C, de Boer RA, et al. How to diagnose heart failure with preserved ejection fraction: the HFA-PEFF diagnostic algorithm: a consensus recommendation from the Heart Failure Association (HFA) of the European Society of Cardiology (ESC). Eur J Heart Fail 2020;22:391–412.
6. Eisman AS, Shah RV, Dhakal BP, et al. Pulmonary capillary wedge pressure patterns during exercise predict exercise capacity and incident heart failure. Circ Heart Fail 2018;11:e004750.
7. Lewis GD, Bossone E, Naeije R, et al. Pulmonary vascular hemodynamic response to exercise in cardiopulmonary diseases. Circulation 2013;128: 1470–9.
8. Reddy YNV, Andersen MJ, Obokata M, et al. Arterial stiffening with exercise in patients with heart failure and preserved ejection fraction. J Am Coll Cardiol 2017;70:136–48.
9. Sorimachi H, Burkhoff D, Verbrugge FH, et al. Obesity, venous capacitance, and venous compliance in heart failure with preserved ejection fraction. Eur J Heart Fail 2021;23:1648–58.
10. Baratto C, Caravita S, Dewachter C, et al. Right heart adaptation to exercise in pulmonary hypertension: an invasive hemodynamic study. J Card Fail 2023;29:1261–72.
11. Dhakal BP, Malhotra R, Murphy RM, et al. Mechanisms of exercise intolerance in heart failure with preserved ejection fraction: the role of abnormal peripheral oxygen extraction. Circ Heart Fail 2015;8: 286–94.
12. Houstis NE, Eisman AS, Pappagianopoulos PP, et al. Exercise intolerance in heart failure with preserved ejection fraction: diagnosing and ranking its causes using personalized O2 pathway analysis. Circulation 2018;137:148–61.
13. Gorter TM, Obokata M, Reddy YNV, et al. Exercise unmasks distinct pathophysiologic features in heart failure with preserved ejection fraction and pulmonary vascular disease. Eur Heart J 2018;39: 2825–35.
14. Borlaug BA, Kane GC, Melenovsky V, et al. Abnormal right ventricular-pulmonary artery coupling with exercise in heart failure with preserved ejection fraction. Eur Heart J 2016;37: 3293–302.

15. Guazzi M, Wilhelm M, Halle M, et al. Exercise testing in heart failure with preserved ejection fraction: an appraisal through diagnosis, pathophysiology and therapy - a clinical consensus statement of the Heart Failure Association and European Association of Preventive Cardiology of the European Society of Cardiology. Eur J Heart Fail 2022;24:1327–45.

16. Bellofiore A, Dinges E, Naeije R, et al. Reduced haemodynamic coupling and exercise are associated with vascular stiffening in pulmonary arterial hypertension. Heart (British Cardiac Society) 2017;103: 421–7.

17. Naeije R, Vanderpool R, Dhakal BP, et al. Exercise-induced pulmonary hypertension: physiological basis and methodological concerns. Am J Respir Crit Care Med 2013;187:576–83.

18. Wang Z, Chesler NC. Pulmonary vascular mechanics: important contributors to the increased right ventricular afterload of pulmonary hypertension. Exp Physiol 2013;98:1267–73.

19. Reeves JT, Linehan JH, Stenmark KR. Distensibility of the normal human lung circulation during exercise. Am J Physiol Lung Cell Mol Physiol 2005;288: L419–25.

20. Argiento P, Vanderpool RR, Mule M, et al. Exercise stress echocardiography of the pulmonary circulation: limits of normal and gender differences. Chest 2012. https://doi.org/10.1378/chest.12-0071.

21. Hsu S, Houston BA, Tampakakis E, et al. Right ventricular functional reserve in pulmonary arterial hypertension. Circulation 2016;133(24):2413–22.

22. Leopold JA, Kawut SM, Aldred MA, et al. Diagnosis and treatment of right heart failure in pulmonary vascular diseases: a national heart, lung, and blood institute workshop. Circulation: Heart Fail 2021;14: e007975.

23. Raza F, Chesler NC. Distensibility, an early disease marker of pulmonary vascular health: ready for clinical application. J Am Heart Assoc 2023;12: e031605.

24. Vanderpool RR, Saul M, Nouraie M, et al. Association between hemodynamic markers of pulmonary hypertension and outcomes in heart failure with preserved ejection fraction. JAMA Cardiology 2018;3: 298.

25. Malhotra R, Dhakal BP, Eisman AS, et al. Pulmonary vascular distensibility predicts pulmonary hypertension severity, exercise capacity, and survival in heart failure. Circulation: Heart Fail 2016;9:e003011.

26. Berry NC, Manyoo A, Oldham WM, et al. Protocol for exercise hemodynamic assessment: performing an invasive cardiopulmonary exercise test in clinical practice. Pulm Circ 2015;5:610–8.

27. Wallace WD, Nouraie M, Chan SY, et al. Treatment of exercise pulmonary hypertension improves pulmonary vascular distensibility. Pulm Circ 2018;8. 2045894018787381.

28. Lau EMT, Iyer N, Ilsar R, et al. Abnormal pulmonary artery stiffness in pulmonary arterial hypertension: in vivo study with intravascular ultrasound. PLoS One 2012;7:e33331.

29. Singh I, Oliveira RKF, Naeije R, et al. Pulmonary vascular distensibility and early pulmonary vascular remodeling in pulmonary hypertension. Chest 2019; 156:724–32.

30. Elliott J, Menakuru N, Martin KJ, et al. iCPET calculator: a web-based application to standardize the calculation of alpha distensibility in patients with pulmonary arterial hypertension. J Am Heart Assoc 2023;12:e029667.

31. Raza F, Kozitza C, Lechuga C, et al. Multimodality deep phenotyping methods to assess mechanisms of poor right ventricular–pulmonary artery coupling. Function (Oxf) 2022;3:zqac022.

32. Sanz J, Sánchez-Quintana D, Bossone E, et al. Anatomy, function, and dysfunction of the right ventricle: JACC state-of-the-art review. J Am Coll Cardiol 2019;73:1463–82.

33. Friedman SH, Tedford RJ. Are you coupled? Hemodynamic phenotyping in pulmonary hypertension. Function (Oxf) 2022;3:zqac036.

34. Tang WHW, Wilcox JD, Jacob MS, et al. Comprehensive diagnostic evaluation of cardiovascular physiology in patients with pulmonary vascular disease: insights from the PVDOMICS program. Circ Heart Fail 2020;13:e006363.

35. Kovacs G, Avian A, Olschewski A, et al. Zero reference level for right heart catheterisation. Eur Respir J 2013;42:1586–94.

36. Campedelli L, Nouraie SM, Risbano MG. Non-arterial line cardiac output calculation misclassifies exercise pulmonary hypertension and increases risk of data loss particularly in black, scleroderma and Raynaud's patients during invasive exercise testing. Eur Respir J 2024;64:2302232.

37. Verwerft J, Bertrand PB, Claessen G, et al. Cardiopulmonary exercise testing with simultaneous echocardiography: blueprints of a dyspnea clinic for suspected HFpEF. JACC Heart Fail 2023;11:243–9.

38. Hubert A, Girerd N, Le Breton H, et al. Diagnostic accuracy of lung ultrasound for identification of elevated left ventricular filling pressure. Int J Cardiol 2019;281:62–8.

39. Pugliese NR, De Biase N, Conte L, et al. Cardiac reserve and exercise capacity: insights from combined cardiopulmonary and exercise echocardiography stress testing. J Am Soc Echocardiogr 2021; 34:38–50.

40. Backhaus SJ, Lange T, George EF, et al. Exercise stress real-time cardiac magnetic resonance imaging for noninvasive characterization of heart failure with preserved ejection fraction: the HFpEF-stress trial. Circulation 2021;143:1484–98.

Cardiopulmonary Exercise Testing, Rehabilitation, and Exercise Training in Postpulmonary Embolism

Naga Dharmavaram, MD[a], Amir Esmaeeli, MD[a], Kurt Jacobson, MD[a], Yevgeniy Brailovsky, DO, MSc[b], Farhan Raza, MD[a],*

KEYWORDS

- Pulmonary embolism • Postpulmonary embolism syndrome • Cardiopulmonary exercise test
- Exercise training • Rehabilitation

KEY POINTS

- Exercise intolerance and functional impairments 3 to 6 months after an acute pulmonary embolism (PE) are common and should be investigated with cardiopulmonary exercise test (CPET).
- If significant CPET abnormalities are detected (reduced peak VO_2, abnormal V_E/VCO_2), further testing should be performed, which includes ventilation perfusion scan for pulmonary vascular occlusion from residual thrombus and echocardiogram for pulmonary hypertension and right heart failure.
- Exercise training and rehabilitation should be discussed and prescribed.
- It remains unclear if treatments beyond anticoagulation, catheter-directed therapies, and thrombolytics affect functional impairments at 3 to 6 months post-PE.

INTRODUCTION

Long-term exercise intolerance and functional limitations are common after an episode of acute pulmonary embolism (PE), despite 3 to 6 months of anticoagulation.[1] These persistent symptoms are reported in more than half of the patients with acute PE and are referred as "post-PE syndrome."[2] Although these functional limitations can occur from persistent pulmonary vascular occlusion or pulmonary vascular remodeling,[3] significant deconditioning can be a major contributing factor.[4] Herein, the authors review the role of exercise testing to elucidate the mechanisms of exercise limitations to guide next steps in management and exercise training for musculoskeletal deconditioning.

POST-PULMONARY EMBOLISM EXERCISE IMPAIRMENT

After an episode of acute PE, anticoagulation for at least 3 months is recommended for most patients with provoked PE (due to an identifiable reversible risk factor, eg, surgery, estrogen use, trauma, and immobility).[5–7] A prolonged and indefinite anticoagulation should be considered in select cases (unprovoked PE, persistent risk factor, recurrent

This article originally appeared in *Interventional Cardiology Clinics*, Volume 12 Issue 3, July 2023.

a Division of Cardiology, Department of Medicine, University of Wisconsin-Madison, Hospitals and Clinics, 600 Highland Avenue CSC-E5/582B, Madison, WI 53792, USA; b Division of Cardiology, Department of Medicine, Jefferson Heart Institute-Sidney Kimmel School of Medicine, Thomas Jefferson University, 111 South 11th Street, Philadelphia, PA 19107, USA

* Corresponding author. University of Wisconsin-Madison, Hospitals and Clinics, 600 Highland Avenue CSC-E5/582B, Madison, WI 53792.

E-mail address: fraza@medicine.wisc.edu

heartfailure.theclinics.com

PE). Most of the clinical improvement and acute clot resolution occurs in the first 3 months,[8,9] and the optimal time to assess residual exercise impairment is 3 to 6 months after the acute PE episode.[4,10,11]

As indicated in **Fig. 1**, there are 3 possible sequalae after treatment of acute PE after 3 to 6 months of anticoagulation. Although most patients have resolution of clot, nearly 30% have residual pulmonary vascular obstruction from chronic thromboembolic disease. Among these patients, some have no resting pulmonary hypertension (chronic thromboembolic disease [CTED]), and others develop chronic thromboembolic pulmonary hypertension (CTEPH, nearly 4% of all patients post-PE).[2,12] As indicated in **Fig. 2**, persistent functional limitations can occur from varying and overlapping causes and should be quantified with exercise testing.[13,14] Additional ancillary testing should be considered with ventilation perfusion (VQ) scan and echocardiogram to assess for persistent perfusion defects, pulmonary hypertension (PH), and right ventricular dysfunction.[4,10,11]

Quality-of-Life Surveys

A variety of quality-of-life (QoL) questionnaires are available to assess functional impairments in patients after acute PE. Besides generic QoL questionnaires, such as the 36-Item Short Form Health Survey (SF-36) and Kansas City Cardiomyopathy Questionnaire (KCCQ), there are PE-specific questionnaires, such as the Pulmonary Embolism Quality of Life Questionnaire (PEmb-QoL). The PEmb-QoL questionnaire is a reliable instrument to assess QoL after acute PE.[15] It includes 9 questions and assesses 6 domains: frequency of complaints, activities of daily living limitations, work-related problems, social limitations, intensity of complaints, and emotional complaints. Higher scores indicate a worse QoL.

The FOCUS (Follow-Up after Acute Pulmonary Embolism) study is a prospective, multicenter trial that followed-up patients for 2 years after the event of an acute PE. The trial assessed QoL measures via the PEmb-QoL questionnaire at 3 and 12 months following acute PE. At the 3-month mark, patients could be divided into tertiles, with 34.4% feeling worse than baseline, 29.9% feeling the same, and 26% feeling better than baseline. At the 12-month mark, 55.4% felt better than baseline, whereas 20.3% had complete resolution of problems/symptoms. The data from the trial showed that at both time points, worse QoL was associated with female sex, elevated body mass index (BMI), and preexisting cardiopulmonary disease.[16]

The ELOPE (Prospective Evaluation of Long-term Outcomes After Pulmonary Embolism) study, examined post-PE effects on dyspnea, QoL, and exercise capacity after treatment with warfarin. The study found that most patients had improvement in these dimensions over 1 year, with the greatest improvement manifesting in the first 3 months after treatment.[9] It also found that female sex, elevated BMI, and poor exercise-capacity measured at 1 month post-PE (defined by percent-predicted oxygen consumption VO_2 less than 80% on cardiopulmonary exercise) was associated with worse outcomes.[17]

A similar study by Josien and colleagues reported that in 109 post-PE patients QoL (per SF-36 and PEmb-QoL surveys at a median follow-up of 25 months post-PE) was reduced and comparable to patients with acute myocardial infarction the previous year.[18] More importantly, the study suggested that higher thrombus load did not seem to affect QoL on the long-term.

Cardiopulmonary Exercise Test

In addition to QoL surveys, a symptom-limited cardiopulmonary exercise testing (CPET) is the best tool to assess functional impairments in various cardiopulmonary diseases.[19–23] It provides diagnostic value in discriminating multisystem contributions in multifactorial dyspnea and prognostic value to determine clinical outcomes.[19,21,24]

A. *CPET metrics*: the methodology and measurements of CPET are described in the ATS/ACCP statement[25] and other detailed reviews.[17,19,26,27] Herein, we present a more simplified stepwise approach as a practical guide to interpreting CPET. (1) *Peak VO_2:* peak VO_2, adjusted for weight (mL/Kg/min) and reported as percentage predicted (based on age and sex), indicates the maximal exercise capacity. Peak VO_2 less than 80% of predicted indicates exercise intolerance in post-PE patients.[23,28] (2) *Respiratory exchange ratio (RER)*: peak exercise RER (carbon dioxide output: VCO_2 to VO_2 ratio), greater than or equal to 1.1 indicates a good effort, RER less than 1.0 indicates a poor, whereas an RER 1.0 to 1.1 indicates a fair effort.[17] An RER less than 1.1 suggests deconditioning and inability to cross anaerobic threshold (AT), albeit coronary artery disease (CAD), and chronic obstructive pulmonary disease (COPD) can also be a major limiting factor.[17,19,25,26] (3) *Gas exchange, V_E/VCO_2:* linking minute ventilation (V_E) to VCO_2 results in matching ventilation-to-perfusion response to exercise and is defined as ventilatory efficiency.[17] V_E/VCO_2 reflects efficiency of alveolar-capillary interface, chemoreceptor sensitivity, and acid-

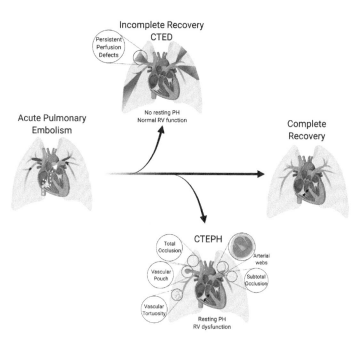

Fig. 1. Sequalae after treatment of acute pulmonary embolism with 3 to 6 months of anticoagulation. CTED, chronic thromboembolic disease; CTEPH, chronic thromboembolic pulmonary hypertension; PH, pulmonary hypertension; RV, right ventricle. (Created in BioRender. Brailovsky, Y. (2021) BioRender.com/t39u676).

base balance. With exercise, there is improved VQ matching and reduction in V_E/VCO_2 till AT is achieved. There is an increase in V_E/VCO_2 after AT due to metabolic acidosis and hyperventilation. Similar to V_E/VCO_2, other metrics of gas exchange improve with exercise: $PETCO_2$ (partial pressure of end-tidal carbon dioxide) increases, and V_D/V_T (physiologic dead-space fraction) decreases.[27] Abnormal V_E/VCO_2 correlates with symptoms and disease severity in cardiopulmonary diseases with V_E/VCO_2 greater than 35 considered a high-risk feature.[17,19,22,25,27,29,30] Zhai and colleagues reported that V_E/VCO_2 (mean value) is worse in CTEPH (51), versus a comparable pulmonary arterial hypertension (PAH) cohort (44) with similar peak VO_2.[31] McCabe and colleagues reported that nadir V_E/VCO_2 at AT (mean value) can differentiate normal subjects (27) from CTED (37) and CTEPH (46).[13] These studies

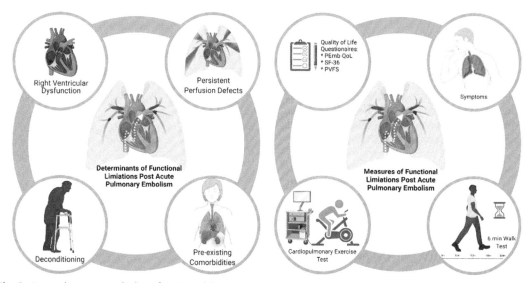

Fig. 2. Postpulmonary embolism functional limitations: quantifying and determining causes. PEmb-QoL, Pulmonary Embolism Quality of Life Questionnaire; PVFS, post-venous thromboembolism functional status; SF-36, 36-Item Short Form Health Survey. (Created in BioRender. Brailovsky, Y. (2021) BioRender.com/t39u676).

indicate the additional burden of poor gas exchange and breathlessness from residual thrombus, even in the absence of pulmonary vascular disease. (4) *Breathing Reserve (BR)*: BR corresponds to ventilatory (lung parenchymal) reserve at peak exercise and is traditionally defined as the percentage of MVV (maximal ventilatory volume = FEV1 x 35–40) achieved at peak exercise ([$V_E$max/MVV] x 100%).[25] A breathing reserve less than 15% to 20% suggests pulmonary disease as a primary cause of dyspnea. However, there is significant reported variance in normal value for BR, and some studies suggesting that BR less than 15% to 20% can underestimate true ventilatory limitation of COPD even with relatively low-intensity exercise.[32] (5) *O_2 pulse*: oxygen pulse (O_2 pulse = VO_2/heart rate) is a reasonable surrogate of stroke volume and indicates cardiac response to exercise (eg, right ventricular limitation to exercise in a post-PE patient). However, O_2 pulse also depends on arteriovenous oxygen difference (O_2 extraction), and different thresholds have not been extensively validated. In a study of patients with heart failure with reduced ejection fraction (HFrEF) (n = 209), Lavie and colleagues reported that an O2 pulse greater than or equal to 10 mL/beat predicted event-free survival on a follow-up of 40 months.[33] (6) *Heart rate*: a normal exercise response requires a nearly 2.2-fold increase in heart rate, and the augmentation of heart rate from rest to exercise is referred as heart rate reserve (HRR).[34] Inability to achieve greater than or equal to 80% of HRR or greater than or equal to 80% of age-predicted maximal heart rate (220-age) indicates chronotropic incompetence (CI).[34,35] CI is identified as a major contributory factor to chronic cardiopulmonary diseases, including post-PE (ELOPE study).[23,34,35] It remains unclear if CI reflects peripheral muscle deconditioning or reduced cardiac beta-receptor sensitivity.[36] However, cardiac rehabilitation has been shown to improve CI in patients with CAD,[37] and 6-minute walk distance in patients with heart failure.[38] Recovery of heart rate after exercise also indicates good cardiovascular health and is defined as decrease in heart rate from peak exercise to 2 minutes of recovery of less than 42 beats per minute.[34,39] (8) *Miscellaneous*: peripheral oxygen desaturation (SpO_2) with exercise is a sign of pulmonary vascular disease such as CTEPH or thromboembolic disease without PH such as CTED.[23,31] Exercise oscillatory ventilation has been described in postcapillary PH, presumed due to stimulation of pulmonary

J-receptors from increase in left-heart filling pressures, but not reported in PAH or thromboembolic disease.[19] Lastly, VO_2 kinetics reveal significant patterns of cardiopulmonary limitations in PH and heart failure,[19,20,40] which are beyond the scope of the current review.

B. *CPET modality: Treadmill versus ergometer*: CPET can be performed with a treadmill or cycle ergometer (upright or recumbent in most noninvasive laboratories). In comparison to cycle ergometer, treadmill CPET results in a higher peak VO_2 due to increased muscle mass recruitment.[25,26] However, cycle ergometer provides significant benefits that include higher safety, less noise, ease of ramp protocol, and blood gas collection.[25,26]

Regarding impact of exercise modality on V_E/VCO_2, Valli and colleagues reported on 13 patients with severe PAH (mean pulmonary artery pressure = 65 mm Hg) undergoing treadmill and ergometer CPETs 24 to 48 hours apart.[41] The study reported a higher V_E/VCO_2 ratio at anaerobic threshold with treadmill (56) versus ergometer (45). Although the sample size was small, the investigators suggested that treadmill test provided a more accurate depiction of VQ abnormalities and disease severity. Based on this study, a treadmill CPET may be better suited for post-PE patients undergoing CPET to identify physiologic dead-space from vascular occlusions.

C. *CPET in cardiopulmonary diseases and post-PE state:* CPET provides significant prognostic information in different cardiopulmonary diseases, as summarized in **Table 1**. More importantly, it can identify burden of cardiopulmonary versus peripheral muscular limitations and guide management steps after 3 to 6 months of anticoagulation in a post-PE patient. In the ELOPE study,[23] reduced exercise capacity was associated with male sex, elevated BMI, and history of smoking. Most (87.5%) of those with diminished exercise capacity were due to physical deconditioning; however, a significant minority (12.5%) were due to ventilatory defects. Subsequent imaging analysis revealed no correlation of residual perfusion defects with reduced peak VO_2.[42] These findings suggest that physical deconditioning is the main cause for residual exercise impairment in post-PE patients. Similar prospective study by Albaghdadi and colleagues in 20 post-PE patients suggests reduced peak VO_2 in 60% patients, predominantly due to deconditioning.[43]

D. *Invasive CPET:* in subjects with exercise impairment and CPET abnormalities, with suspected CTED or CTEPH, an invasive CPET can confirm

Table 1
Major cardiopulmonary exercise studies in different cardiopulmonary diseases

Study	Details	Modality	Major Findings
HFrEF Mancini DM, et al,[21] 1991	Prospective N = 122, mean age = 50 y, 15% women	Treadmill	Three subgroups: 1. Peak VO_2 > 14 mL/Kg/min (n = 52) had 94% 1-y survival 2. Peak VO_2 < 14 mL/Kg/min (n = 27) and not transplant candidates had 47% 1-y survival 3. Peak VO_2 < 14 mL/Kg/min (n = 35) and awaiting transplant had 70% 1-y survival
HFrEF Osman AF, et al,[44] 2000	Prospective N = 225, mean age = 54 y, 20% women	Treadmill	Peak VO_2 mL/Kg/min <19 per lean body mass is superior to peak VO_2 < 14 in predicting outcomes Percent fat = 25.9% in the cohort, and 37% subjects had BMI $\geq$30 kg/m^2
HFrEF Arena R, et al,[29] 2007	Prospective N = 448, mean age = 57 y, 21% women	Treadmill	Based on V_E/VCO_2, 4 groups were defined: (i) $\leq$29, (ii) 30–35.9, (iii) 36–44.9, (iv) $\geq$45.0 and had respectively predictive event-free survival at 2 y: 97%, 85%, 72%, and 44%
PAH Yasunobu, et al,[45] 2005	Retrospective N = 52 (control = 9), mean age = 44 y, 86% women	Cycle ergometer	Four PAH subgroups per peak VO_2 %-predicted (mild: 65%–79%; moderate: 50%–64%; severe: 35%–49%; very severe: 35%), control = 93% 1. V_E/VCO_2 ratio at AT significantly higher in all PAH subgroups (37, 42, 45, 67), control = 27 2. $PETCO_2$ (mm Hg) at AT was lower in all PAH subgroups (33, 28, 26, and 18), control = 42

(continued on next page)

Table 1
(continued)

Study	Details	Modality	Major Findings
PAH Sun, et al,[46] 2001	Retrospective N = 53 (20 controls), mean age = 42 y, 88% women	Cycle ergometer	V_E/VCO_2 slope was significantly higher in PAH subjects (47) compared with controls (25) Peak VO_2 (mL/kg/min) was significantly lower in PAH (12) compared with controls (30)
HFpEF Dhakal, et al,[47] 2015	Prospective N = 48 (controls = 24), mean age = 63 y, women = 60%	Invasive CPET with upright cycle ergometer	Peak VO_2 (mL/kg/min) = 13.9 (27.0 in controls) Impaired peripheral oxygen extraction (C[a-v]O_2 = 11.5 mL/dL vs 13.3 mL/dL in controls) and reduced peak heart rate (121 vs 148 in controls)
CTEPH Zhai, et al,[31] 2011	Retrospective N = 50 (PAH = 77), mean age = 60 y, women = 46%	Cycle ergometer	Worse dead space ventilation in CTEPH: V_E/VCO_2 slope = 51 (44 in PAH), despite similar peak VO_2 (mL/kg/min) 13.8 in CTEPH, vs 14.5 in PAH.
Post-PE ELOPE study Kahn SR, et al,[23] 2017	Prospective N = 100, mean age = 50 y, 43% women	Cycle ergometer	46.5% patients had peak VO_2 <80% predicted (n = 86 pts completed 1-y follow-up) Reduced peak VO_2 attributed to deconditioning; not predicted by residual thrombus on repeat imaging.[42]
Post-PE Albaghdadi Mazen S, et al,[43] 2018	Prospective N = 20, mean age = 57 y, 40% women	Cycle ergometer	12/20 (60%) with peak VO_2 <80% at 6-mo. Deconditioning suggested as predominant cause of persistent dyspnea

Abbreviations: AT, anaerobic threshold; BMI, body mass index; C[a-v]O2, arteriovenous oxygen concentration difference; CTEPH, chronic thromboembolic pulmonary hypertension; HFpEF, heart failure with preserved ejection fraction; HFrEF, heart failure with reduced ejection fraction; PAH, pulmonary arterial hypertension; PETCO2, partial pressure of end-tidal carbon dioxide; VE/VCO2, minute ventilation to carbon dioxide production; VO2, oxygen consumption.

the diagnosis and guide PAH vasodilator therapies. A cycle ergometer is used for invasive CPET studies either in an upright, supine, or recumbent position.

The detailed methods are described by expert centers.[48–52] Briefly, a right internal jugular venous access for a pulmonary arterial catheter and a right radial cannula for arterial monitoring is placed. Ramp protocol on a cycle ergometer is used for rest-to-exercise invasive CPET study, along with a metabolic cart (**Figs. 3** and **4**). Pressure flow (direct Fick cardiac output) measurements are acquired during different stages of exercise. A

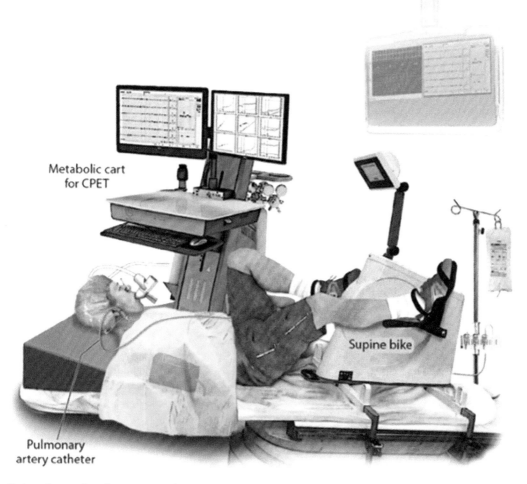

Fig. 3. Invasive cardiopulmonary exercise test.

lactate level is checked at peak exercise to confirm elevated level and adequacy of effort. Based on established criteria for exercise PH,[4,49,53,54] the hemodynamic diagnosis of post-PE patients is confirmed as CTED or CTEPH. These criteria include mean pulmonary artery pressure/cardiac output slope greater than or equal to 3 mm Hg/L/min[49] and peak exercise transpulmonary resistance greater than or equal to 3 mm Hg/L/min.[53]

Six-Minute Walk Test

Six-minute walk test (6MWT) is a simple and reproducible tool to assess functional limitations.[55–57] It has been extensively used in clinical trials, and its correlation with CPET metrics and NYHA class has been reported.[58] Miyamoto and colleagues reported a study of 43 PAH patients undergoing 6MWT and CPET. Walk distance in NYHA classes (2/3/4) was ~440, 320, and 100 m. Median 6MWT of 332 m predicted clinical outcomes on 5-year

follow-up. 6MWT correlated modestly with cardiac output ($r = 0.48$, $P < .05$) and total pulmonary resistance ($r = -0.49$, $P < .05$) and strongly with peak VO_2 ($r = 0.70$, $P < .001$), and V_E/VCO_2 slope ($r = -0.66$, $P < .001$). 6MWT is a useful tool in centers that lack CPET facilities.

EXERCISE TRAINING IN CARDIOPULMONARY DISEASE

Peripheral muscle deconditioning is present in nearly half post-PE patients.[23,59] These limitations are reported even after receiving thrombolytics (PEITHO trial),[60] whereas more studies are needed to assess long-term limitations in patients receiving catheter-directed thrombolytics for acute PE.[61–64] To address the deconditioning, pulmonary and cardiac rehabilitation have been a mainstay in the treatment of PAH, HFrEF, HFpEF (heart failure with preserved ejection fraction), and COPD in helping increase exercise capacity and various

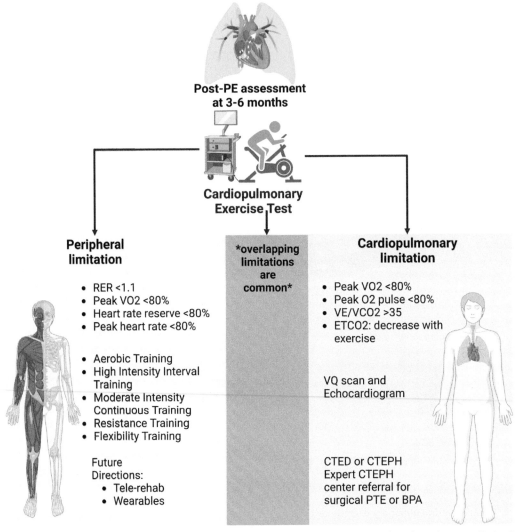

Fig. 4. Algorithm for post-PE follow-up. *, combination of peripheral limitation and cardiopulmonary limitation. BPA, balloon pulmonary angioplasty; CTED, chronic thromboembolic disease; CTEPH, chronic thromboembolic pulmonary hypertension; ETCO₂, end-tidal carbon dioxide pressure; O₂ pulse, oxygen pulse (VO₂/heart rate); PE, pulmonary embolism; RER, respiratory exchange ratio; V$_E$/VCO₂, minute ventilation to carbon dioxide output ratio; VO₂, oxygen consumption; VQ, ventilation-perfusion. (Created in BioRender. Brailovsky, Y. (2021) BioRender.com/t39u676).

aspects of psychosomatic health.[65–67] These chronic conditions produce skeletal muscle alterations, detraining, and deconditioning.[68] Further, Lowe and colleagues have shown that a reduction in exercise capacity in the setting of PH has been associated with depression and anxiety.[69]

In post-PE patients, early participation in exercise and structured rehabilitation programs have been found safe and effective in multiple studies (**Table 2**).[70–73] In some studies, exercise regimen was started as early as 1-month post-PE.[72,80] Although in-person pulmonary rehabilitation has been used in most studies, remote home-based

regimen has been reported to be efficacious for post-PE patients,[72] similar to CAD and heart failure.[77,81] Hence for post-PE patients, the American Physical Therapy Association has published guidelines for physical therapist to implement exercise regimen after an episode of thromboembolic disease.[82]

Exercise Goals

The goals of a cardiac rehabilitation program are to assess a patient's baseline ability and limitations, develop an exercise prescription, observe the

Table 2
Major studies on rehabilitation and structured exercise programs in postpulmonary embolism and other cardiopulmonary diseases

Study Name	Disease	Type of Exercise Regimen	Modality of Exercise	Frequency of Exercise	Duration of Exercise	Major Outcomes/ Findings
PeRehab Study Haukeland-Parker, et al,[70] 2021	Post-PE	Outpatient rehabilitation vs usual care	Interval and resistance training	2x per wk	8 wk	Ongoing trial n = 190, 1:1 randomization
Pulmonary rehabilitation post-PE and cardiac MRI Gleditsch, et al,[71] 2022	Post-PE	Outpatient rehabilitation vs usual care	Supervised resistance and endurance training	2x per wk	8 wk	n = 26, significant improvement in "Shortness of Breath Questionnaire" (median 15–8) and reduction in right ventricular mass (49–44 g)
Physiotherapist-guided home-based exercise Rolving et al,[72] 2020	Post-PE	Home-based vs usual care	Variable (patient-preferred exercise modality)	3x per wk	8 wk	n = 140 with 1:1 randomization and exercise regimen 1–3 mo post-PE. Exercise was safe Improvement in incremental shuttle walk test on 6-mo follow-up: 104 vs 78 m (P = .27)
Pulmonary rehabilitation post-PE Nopp et al,[73] 2020	Post-PE	Single-arm intervention	Cycle ergometer, inspiratory muscle training	3x per wk	6 wk	n = 22, rehabilitation started 19 wk post-PE 6MWD improved by 49.4 m on completion

(continued on next page)

Table 2
(continued)

Study Name	Disease	Type of Exercise Regimen	Modality of Exercise	Frequency of Exercise	Duration of Exercise	Major Outcomes/ Findings
Fox et al,[74] 2011	PAH, CTEPH	6 wk HIIT and 6 wk MICT	Treadmill, cycling, step climbing, resistance training	24 1-h sessions	12 wk	Increase in 6MWD by 32 m and VO_2Max by 1.1 mL kg^{-1} min^{-1}. No serious adverse events
HF-ACTION O'Connor et al.[75] 2009	Chronic heart failure	Exercise training vs usual care	Cycle or treadmill	3x per wk	12 wk	11% reduction in all-cause mortality/ hospitalizations and a 13% reduction in cardiovascular mortality or heart failure hospitalizations
SAINTEX-CAD Conraads et al,[76] 2015	Coronary artery disease	In-person rehab	HIIT vs MICT	3x per wk	12 wk	Both interval and continuous training improve VO_2Max (22.7 vs 20.3 mL kg^{-1} min^{-1}) at 12 wk and this is sustained at 1 y
REMOTE-CR Maddison et al,[77] 2019	Coronary heart disease	Telerehab vs in-person rehab	Individualized to each participant	3x per wk	12 wk	Peak VO_2 was noninferior; telerehab less sedentary at 24 wk; per capita program delivery and medication costs lower for telerehab

Yoga-CaRe Prabhakaran et al,[78] 2020	Acute myocardial infarction	Yoga vs standard care	Yoga	13 sessions in 12 wk	12 wk	Yoga improved self-rated health and return to preinfarct activities
Ries et al,[79] 2005	COPD	Walking	Pulmonary rehabilitation	Twice daily for 30 min	8 wk	Pulmonary rehab in COPD associated with increased exercise tolerance (1.5 METS vs 0.6 METS)

Abbreviations: 6MWD, 6-minute walk distance; COPD, chronic obstructive pulmonary disease; CTEPH, chronic thromboembolic pulmonary hypertension; HIIT, high-intensity interval training; LVEDD, left ventricular end diastolic volume; MICT, moderate-intensity continuous training; PAH, pulmonary arterial hypertension; PE, pulmonary embolism; VO$_2$Max, maximal oxygen consumption.

patient's response to that prescription, and encourage long-term participation in regular unsupervised exercise. Through these 4 goals, the goal of increasing the patient's cardiorespiratory fitness can be achieved.[83] Additional components of a successful rehabilitation program include psychosocial support, nutritional counseling, weight management, and education regarding diet and medications adherence. All these nonexercise goals further bolster the efficacy of a rehabilitation program[84] and improve patient's cardiorespiratory fitness.

For the best balance of recruiting large muscle groups while still avoiding a higher risk of physical injury, low-impact, aerobic exercises are preferred for a rehabilitation program. Examples include walking, jogging, cycling, rowing, or machine stair climbing.[85] It is important, however, to individualize the exercise regimen to the individual as to promote maximum compliance and reduce risk of injury. To engage the individual, several different types of exercise routines have been studied.

Exercise Modalities

A. *Aerobic exercise training*: aerobic exercise training has been the mainstay of cardiac rehabilitation. Saltin and colleagues demonstrated in 1968 the benefits of exercise in the Dallas Bed Rest and Exercise study,[86] and it was Braunwald, Sarnoff, Sonnenblick, Hellerstein, and Naughton, among others who helped lay the foundation for the present-day cardiac rehabilitation program.[87,88] Twenty percent reduction in all-cause mortality has been observed for each metabolic equivalent improvement in fitness in those with cardiovascular disease.[89]

B. *Moderate intensity continuous training (MICT)*: based on current consensus, MICT consists of aerobic activity that falls within the 60% of maximal heart rate or a 12 to 13 on the Borg scale.[90] MICT has been reported to achieve an increase in the peak VO_2.[90–92]

C. *High-intensity interval training (HIIT)*: recent research has shown that higher intensity exercise leads to greater improvements in peak VO_2 than moderate- or low-intensity exercise. Taylor and colleagues reported a 10% increase in peak VO_2 with HIIT versus a 4% with MICT in patients with CAD.[93] HIIT has been shown to significantly improve respiratory muscle function, ventilatory drive, lung diffusion, and alveolar-capillary conductance, which all contributed to a higher peak VO_2.[94–96] Peripheral vascular adaptations with HIIT include increases in mean blood flow through increases in shear stress stimulus and upregulation of vasodilatory mechanisms, leading to improved endothelial function and flow-mediated dilation, eventually leading to increased peak VO_2.[97–100] Lastly, improved oxidative capacity and mitochondrial adaptations in skeletal muscles enhance O_2 extraction and utilization.[101–103]

D. *Resistance training*: resistance training is an important and safe component of rehabilitation.[104,105] Ozaki and colleagues reported that older patients with a low baseline peak VO_2 (<25 mL kg^{-1} min^{-1}) benefited more from resistance training than those with a higher baseline peak VO_2 (>32 mL kg^{-1} min^{-1}).[106] Hence, sicker patients stand to benefit the most from resistance training.

E. *Flexibility training: Yoga and Tai Chi*: Yoga-CaRe study evaluated the benefit of yoga in cardiac rehabilitation for patients with recent acute myocardial infarction. Although it did not have enough power to show a statistically significant difference in major adverse cardiovascular events, it improved self-rated health and return to preinfarct activities.[78] Liu and colleagues studied Tai chi (another low-impact and low-intensity exercise), and found it to improve aerobic endurance and psychosocial well-being in those with CAD.[107]

Exercise Dose: Frequency, Intensity, and Duration

A rehabilitation program will typically include 3 times a week session for 8 to 12 weeks. A typical rehabilitation session starts with a 5- to 10-minute warm up, followed by 20 to 45 minutes of aerobic activity, and concluded by a 5- to 10-minute cool down. The intensity of exercise ranges from 40% to 85% of peak VO_2 (55%–90% of maximal heart rate [HR] = 220-age). The intensity of exercise based on maximal heart rate is characterized as follows:

a Light exercise: <60% of max HR
b Moderate exercise: 60% to 79% of max HR
c Heavy exercise: ≥80% of max HR

Another measure of exertion that is commonly used in rehabilitation programs is the "rating of perceived exertion" (RPE) on the Borg scale. The scale is measured from 6 to 20 and an RPE of 12 to 13 is perceived to be "somewhat hard," which should correlate to 60% of the peak VO2, and an RPE of 16 is perceived to be "hard-to-very hard," which correlates to 85% of peak VO2.[108] Based on these studies, an individualized light-to-moderate exercise regimen should be routinely prescribed in patients with functional impairments due to muscle deconditioning at 3 months post-PE; this is supported by the 2019 combined guidelines by the European Society of Cardiology and the European Respiratory Society.[109]

Synergy Between Exercise and Medical Interventions

Post-PE cardiopulmonary limitations include residual clot, PAH, right heart dysfunction, and previously undiagnosed left heart disease (CAD, HFpEF). It is essential to have a synergy of prompt management of cardiopulmonary limitations, as the exercise therapies are used.

Although studying the individualized benefit of exercise regimen versus cardiopulmonary intervention is difficult, the exercise regimen is proved to improve the overall health of any patient with a cardiopulmonary comorbidity.[110,111]

Future Directions: Telerehabilitation and Wearables

Technology-assisted delivery methods (telerehabilitation) can overcome significant barriers of health care accessibility and lower costs. REMOTE-CR trial of 162 patients with CAD, delivered remotely monitored telerehabilitation (n = 82) and center-based rehabilitation (n = 80).[112] Telerehabilitation delivery (vs in-person rehabilitation) was equally effective (peak VO_2 at 12-week: 30.5 vs 29.4 mL/Kg/min), with significantly lower costs.[77] Future studies are needed to validate these findings in patients after acute PE. With the advent of wearable health monitoring devices such as the Apple Watch, WHOOP, Garmin, and Fitbit, there has been a renewed interest in incorporating them into the cardiac rehabilitation world. In addition, given the relative equivalence of remote versus center-based delivery of rehabilitation services, these devices could be a paradigm shift in the concept of cardiac rehabilitation.[113,114] Given the COVID-19 pandemic and the costs associated with traveling to a center-based program, wearable-assisted home programs could further enhance participation and long-term compliance.

SUMMARY

After 3 to 6 months of anticoagulation for acute PE, residual functional impairments and exercise intolerance are present in more than half of the patients. Although residual thromboembolic burden exists in nearly one-third cases, deconditioning contributes to exercise impairment in nearly all these patients. Different modality and delivery methods of structured exercise regimen should be used for long-term improvements in exercise capacity and quality of life.

CLINICS CARE POINTS

- In assessing a patient at 3-months after an acute PE episode, assess residual exercise intolerance with history and consider a cardiopulmonary exercise test to objectify.

- If persistent dyspnea or CPET abnormalities exist, consider a VQ scan and echocardiogram.

- For peripheral muscle deconditioning, prescribe structured exercise regimen.

ACKNOWLEDGMENTS

None.

REFERENCES

1. Klok FA, Tijmensen JE, Haeck MLA, et al. Persistent dyspnea complaints at long-term follow-up after an episode of acute pulmonary embolism: Results of a questionnaire. Eur J Intern Med 2008;19(8):625–9.

2. Klok FA, van der Hulle T, den Exter PL, et al. The post-PE syndrome: A new concept for chronic complications of pulmonary embolism. Blood Rev 2014;28(6):221–6.

3. Nijkeuter M, Hovens MMC, Davidson BL, et al. Resolution of thromboemboli in patients with acute pulmonary embolism: A systematic review. Chest 2006;129(1):192–7.

4. Morris TA, Timothy M, Fernandes RC. How we do it: evaluation of dyspnea and exercise intolerance after acute pulmonary embolism. Chest 2022. S0012-3692(22)01215-01216.

5. Prediletto R, Paoletti P, Fornai E, et al. Natural course of treated pulmonary embolism. Evaluation by perfusion lung scintigraphy, gas exchange, and chest roentgenogram. Chest 1990;97(3):554–61.

6. Baglin T, Bauer K, Douketis J, et al. Duration of anticoagulant therapy after a first episode of an unprovoked pulmonary embolus or deep vein thrombosis: Guidance from the SSC of the ISTH. J Thromb Haemost 2012;10(4):698–702.

7. Kearon C, Akl EA, Comerota AJ, et al. Antithrombotic therapy for VTE disease: Antithrombotic therapy and prevention of thrombosis, 9th ed: American College of Chest Physicians evidence-

based clinical practice guidelines. Chest 2012; 141(2 SUPPL):e419S–96S.

8. Van Es J, Douma RA, Kamphuisen PW, et al. Clot resolution after 3 weeks of anticoagulant treatment for pulmonary embolism: Comparison of computed tomography and perfusion scintigraphy. J Thromb Haemost 2013;11(4):679–85.

9. Kahn SR, Akaberi A, Granton JT, et al. Quality of Life, Dyspnea, and Functional Exercise Capacity Following a First Episode of Pulmonary Embolism: Results of the ELOPE Cohort Study. Am J Med 2017;130(8):990.

10. Boon GJAM, Bogaard HJ, Klok FA. Essential aspects of the follow-up after acute pulmonary embolism: An illustrated review. Res Pract Thromb Haemost 2020;4(6):958–68.

11. Pugliese SC, Kawut SM. The post-pulmonary embolism syndrome: Real or ruse? Ann Am Thorac Soc 2019;16(7):811–4.

12. Pengo V, Lensing AWA, Prins MH, et al. Incidence of Chronic Thromboembolic Pulmonary Hypertension after Pulmonary Embolism. N Engl J Med 2004;350(22):2257–64.

13. Mccabe C, Deboeck G, Harvey I, et al. Inef fi cient exercise gas exchange identi fi es pulmonary hypertension in chronic thromboembolic obstruction following pulmonary embolism. Thromb Res 2013; 132(6):659–65.

14. Topilsky Y, Hayes CL, Khanna AD, et al. Cardiopulmonary exercise test in patients with subacute pulmonary emboli. Heart & Lung J Acute Crit Care 2012;41(2):125–36.

15. Klok FA, Cohn DM, Middeldorp S, et al. Quality of life after pulmonary embolism: validation of the PEmb-QoL Questionnaire. J Thromb Haemost 2010;8(3):523–32.

16. Valerio L, Barco S, Jankowski M, et al. Quality of life 3 and 12 months following acute pulmonary embolism: analysis from a prospective multicenter cohort study. Chest 2021;159(6):2428–38.

17. Milani RV, Lavie CJ, Mehra MR, et al. Understanding the basics of cardiopulmonary exercise testing. Mayo Clin Proc 2006;81(12):1603–11.

18. Josien vE, Paul L den, Kaptein A, et al. Quality of life after pulmonary embolism as assessed with SF-36 and PEmb-QoL. Thromb Res 2013;132(5): 500–5.

19. Malhotra R, Bakken K, D'Elia E, et al. Cardiopulmonary Exercise Testing in Heart Failure. JACC Hear Fail 2016. https://doi.org/10.1016/j.jchf.2016.03.022.

20. Chatterjee NA, Murphy RM, Malhotra R, et al. Prolonged mean vo2 response time in systolic heart failure an indicator of impaired right ventricular-pulmonary vascular function. Circ Hear Fail 2013; 6(3):499–507.

21. Mancini DM, Eisen H, Kussmaul W, et al. Value of peak exercise oxygen consumption for optimal

timing of cardiac transplantation in ambulatory patients with heart failure. Circulation 1991;83(3): 778–86.

22. Weatherald J, Farina S, Bruno N, et al. Cardiopulmonary exercise testing in pulmonary hypertension. Annals of the American Thoracic Society 2017;14(Supplement_1):S84–92.

23. Kahn SR, Hirsch AM, Akaberi A, et al. Functional and Exercise Limitations After a First Episode of Pulmonary Embolism: Results of the ELOPE Prospective Cohort Study. Chest 2017;151(5):1058–68.

24. Popovic D, Arena R, Guazzi M. A flattening oxygen consumption trajectory phenotypes disease severity and poor prognosis in patients with heart failure with reduced, mid-range, and preserved ejection fraction. Eur J Heart Fail 2018;20(7): 1115–24.

25. Weisman IM, Weisman IM, Marciniuk D, et al. ATS/ACCP Statement on cardiopulmonary exercise testing. Am J Respir Crit Care Med 2003;167(2): 211–77.

26. Mezzani A. Cardiopulmonary exercise testing: Basics of methodology and measurements. Ann Am Thorac Soc 2017;14:S3–11.

27. Arena R, Guazzi M, Myers J, et al. Cardiopulmonary exercise testing in the assessment of pulmonary hypertension. Expert Rev Respir Med 2011. https://doi.org/10.1586/ers.11.4.

28. Kahn SR, Hirsch A, Beddaoui M, et al. Post-Pulmonary Embolism Syndrome" after a First Episode of PE: Results of the E.L.O.P.E. Study. Blood 2015; 126(23):650.

29. Arena R, Myers J, Abella J, et al. Development of a ventilatory classification system in patients with heart failure. Circulation 2007;115(18):2410–7.

30. Al JWET, Weatherald J, Philipenko B, et al. Ventilatory efficiency in pulmonary vascular diseases. Eur Respir Rev 2021;30(161):200214.

31. Zhai Z, Murphy K, Tighe H, et al. Differences in ventilatory inefficiency between pulmonary arterial hypertension and chronic thromboembolic pulmonary hypertension. Chest 2011;140(5):1284–91.

32. O'Donnell DE, Elbehairy AF, Faisal A, et al. Exertional dyspnoea in COPD: The clinical utility of cardiopulmonary exercise testing. Eur Respir Rev 2016;25(141):333–47.

33. Lavie CJ, Milani RV, Mehra MR. Peak exercise oxygen pulse and prognosis in chronic heart failure. Am J Cardiol 2004;93(5):588–93.

34. Brubaker PH, Kitzman DW. Chronotropic incompetence: Causes, consequences, and management. Circulation 2011;123(9):1010–20.

35. Zweerink A, van der Lingen ALCJ, Handoko ML, et al. Chronotropic Incompetence in Chronic Heart Failure. Circ Heart Fail 2018;11(8):e004969.

36. Sarma S, Stoller D, Hendrix J, et al. Mechanisms of chronotropic incompetence in heart failure with

preserved ejection fraction. Circ Hear Fail 2020; 1–9. https://doi.org/10.1161/CIRCHEARTFAILURE. 119.006331.

37. Pimenta T, Rocha JA. Cardiac rehabilitation and improvement of chronotropic incompetence: Is it the exercise or just the beta blockers? Rev Port Cardiol 2021;40(12):947–53.

38. Mentz RJ, Whellan DJ, Reeves GR, et al. Rehabilitation Intervention in Older Patients With Acute Heart Failure With Preserved Versus Reduced Ejection Fraction. JACC Hear Fail 2021;9(10): 747–57.

39. Cole CR, Foody JAM, Blackstone EH, et al. Heart rate recovery after submaximal exercise testing as a predictor of mortality in a cardiovascularly healthy cohort. Ann Intern Med 2000;132(7):552–5.

40. Bailey CS, Wooster LT, Buswell M, et al. Post-Exercise Oxygen Uptake Recovery Delay: A Novel Index of Impaired Cardiac Reserve Capacity in Heart Failure. JACC Hear Fail 2018;6(4):329–39.

41. Valli G, Vizza CD, Onorati P, et al. Pathophysiological adaptations to walking and cycling in primary pulmonary hypertension. Eur J Appl Physiol 2008. https://doi.org/10.1007/s00421-007-0600-y.

42. Ma KA, Kahn SR, Akaberi A, et al. Serial imaging after pulmonary embolism and correlation with functional limitation at 12 months: Results of the ELOPE Study. Res Pract Thromb Haemost 2018; 2(4):670–7.

43. Albaghdadi MS, Dudzinski DM, Giordano N, et al. Cardiopulmonary exercise testing in patients following massive and submassive pulmonary embolism. J Am Heart Assoc 2018;7(5):12–4.

44. Osman AF, Mehra MR, Lavie CJ, et al. The incremental prognostic importance of body fat adjusted peak oxygen consumption in chronic heart failure. J Am Coll Cardiol 2000;36(7):2126–31.

45. Yasunobu Y, Oudiz RJ, Sun XG, et al. End-tidal Pco_2 abnormality and exercise limitation in patients with primary pulmonary hypertension. Chest 2005; 127(5):1637–46.

46. Sun Xing-Guo, James E, Hansen RJO, et al. Exercise Pathophysiology in Patients With Primary Pulmonary Hypertension. Circulation 2001;104:429–35.

47. Dhakal BP, Malhotra R, Murphy RM, et al. Mechanisms of exercise intolerance in heart failure with preserved ejection fraction: The role of abnormal peripheral oxygen extraction. Circ Hear Fail 2015; 8(2):286–94.

48. Jain CC, Borlaug BA. Performance and Interpretation of Invasive Hemodynamic Exercise Testing. Chest 2020;158(5):2119–29.

49. Lewis GD, Bossone E, Naeije R, et al. Pulmonary vascular hemodynamic response to exercise in cardiopulmonary diseases. Circulation 2013;128(13):1470–9.

50. Raza F, Kozitza C, Lechuga C, et al. Multimodality deep phenotyping methods to assess mechanisms of poor right ventricular-pulmonary artery coupling. Function 2022;3(4):zqac022.

51. Raza F, Dharmavaram N, Hess T, et al. Distinguishing exercise intolerance in early-stage pulmonary hypertension with invasive exercise hemodynamics: Rest V E/V CO 2 and ETCO 2 identify pulmonary vascular disease. Clin Cardiol 2022;45(7): 742–51.

52. Kozitza CJ, Tao R. Pulmonary vascular distensibility with passive leg raise is comparable to exercise and predictive of clinical outcomes in pulmonary hypertension. Pulm Circ 2022;12(1):e12029.

53. Kovacs G, Herve P, Barbera JA, et al. An official European Respiratory Society statement: pulmonary haemodynamics during exercise. Eur Respir J 2017;50(5). https://doi.org/10.1183/13993003. 00578-2017.

54. Eisman AS, Shah RV, Dhakal BP, et al. Pulmonary Capillary Wedge Pressure Patterns During Exercise Predict Exercise Capacity and Incident Heart Failure. Circ Heart Fail 2018;11(5):e004750.

55. Enright PL. The Six-Minute Walk Test Introduction Standards and Indications 6-Minute Walk Test Versus Shuttle Walk Test Safety Variables Measured Conducting the Test Ensuring Quality Factors That Influence 6-Minute Walk Distance Interpreting the Results Improving the. Respir Care 2003;48(8):783–5. Available at: http://rc.rcjournal. com/content/respcare/48/8/783.full.pdf.

56. Holland AE, Spruit MA, Troosters T, et al. An official European respiratory society/American thoracic society technical standard: Field walking tests in chronic respiratory disease. Eur Respir J 2014; 44(6):1428–46.

57. Singh SJ, Puhan MA, Andrianopoulos V, et al. An official systematic review of the European Respiratory Society/American Thoracic Society: Measurement properties of field walking tests in chronic respiratory disease. Eur Respir J 2014;44(6): 1447–78.

58. Miyamoto S, Nagaya N, Satoh T, et al. Clinical correlates and prognostic significance of six-minute walk test in patients with primary pulmonary hypertension: Comparison with cardiopulmonary exercise testing. Am J Respir Crit Care Med 2000; 161(2 I):487–92.

59. Albaghdadi MS, Dudzinski DM, Giordano N, et al. Cardiopulmonary Exercise Testing in Patients Following Massive and Submassive Pulmonary Embolism. J Am Hear Assoc 2018;7(5). https:// doi.org/10.1161/JAHA.117.006841.

60. Konstantinides SV, Vicaut E, Danays T, et al. Impact of Thrombolytic Therapy on the Long-Term Outcome of Intermediate-Risk Pulmonary Embolism. J Am Coll Cardiol 2017;69(12):1536–44.

61. Lewis AE, Gerstein NS, Venkataramani R. Evolving management trends and outcomes in catheter

management of acute pulmonary embolism. J Cardiothorac Vasc Anesth 2022;36(8 Pt B): 3344–56.

62. Piazza G, Hohlfelder B, Harm PD, et al. A prospective, single-arm, multicenter trial of ultrasound-facilitated, catheter-directed, low-dose fibrinolysis for acute massive and submassive pulmonary embolism: the SEATTLE II study. JACC Cardiovasc Interv 2015; 8(10):1382–92.

63. Kuo WT, Banerjee A, Kim PS, et al. Pulmonary embolism response to fragmentation, embolectomy, and catheter thrombolysis (PERFECT): Initial results from a prospective multicenter registry. Chest 2015;148(3):667–73.

64. Kucher N, Boekstegers P, Müller OJ, et al. Randomized, controlled trial of ultrasound-assisted catheter-directed thrombolysis for acute intermediate-risk pulmonary embolism. Circulation 2014;129(4): 479–86.

65. Sahni S, Capozzi B, Iftikhar A, et al. Pulmonary rehabilitation and exercise in pulmonary arterial hypertension: An underutilized intervention. J Exerc Rehabil 2015;11(2):74–9.

66. Pandey A, Parashar A, Kumbhani D, et al. Exercise training in patients with heart failure and preserved ejection fraction: meta-analysis of randomized control trials. Circ Hear Fail 2015;8(1):33–40.

67. Group CW. Pulmonary rehabilitation for patients with chronic pulmonary disease (COPD): An evidence-based analysis. Ont Health Technol Assess Ser 2012;12(6):1–75.

68. Rehn TA, Munkvik M, Lunde PK, et al. Intrinsic skeletal muscle alterations in chronic heart failure patients: a disease-specific myopathy or a result of deconditioning? Hear Fail Rev 2012;17(3):421–36.

69. Löwe B, Gräfe K, Ufer C, et al. Anxiety and depression in patients with pulmonary hypertension. Psychosom Med 2004;66(6):831–6.

70. Haukeland-Parker S, Jervan O, Johannessen HH, et al. Pulmonary rehabilitation to improve physical capacity, dyspnea, and quality of life following pulmonary embolism (the PeRehab study): study protocol for a two-center randomized controlled trial. Trials 2021;22(1):1–9.

71. Gleditsch J, Jervan, Haukeland-Parker S, et al. Effects of pulmonary rehabilitation on cardiac magnetic resonance parameters in patients with persistent dyspnea following pulmonary embolism. IJC Hear Vasc 2022;40(March):100995.

72. Rolving N, Brocki BC, Bloch-Nielsen JR, et al. Effect of a physiotherapist-guided home-based exercise intervention on physical capacity and patient-reported outcomes among patients with acute pulmonary embolism: a randomized clinical trial. JAMA Netw Open 2020;3(2):e200064.

73. Nopp S, Klok FA, Moik F, et al. Outpatient pulmonary rehabilitation in patients with persisting

symptoms after pulmonary embolism. J Clin Med 2020;9(6):1–12.

74. Fox BD, Kassirer M, Weiss I, et al. Ambulatory rehabilitation improves exercise capacity in patients with pulmonary hypertension. J Card Fail 2011;17(3):196–200.

75. O'Connor CM, Whellan DJ, Lee KL, et al. Efficacy and safety of exercise training in patients with chronic heart failure: HF-ACTION randomized controlled trial. JAMA 2009;301(14):1439–50.

76. Conraads VM, Pattyn N, De Maeyer C, et al. Aerobic interval training and continuous training equally improve aerobic exercise capacity in patients with coronary artery disease: The SAINTEX-CAD study. Int J Cardiol 2015;179:203–10.

77. Maddison R, Rawstorn JC, Stewart RAH, et al. Effects and costs of real-time cardiac telerehabilitation: Randomised controlled non-inferiority trial. Heart 2019;105(2):122–9.

78. Prabhakaran D, Chandrasekaran AM, Singh K, et al. Yoga-based cardiac rehabilitation after acute myocardial infarction: a randomized trial. J Am Coll Cardiol 2020;75(13):1551–61.

79. Ries AL, Make BJ, Lee SM, et al. The effects of pulmonary rehabilitation in the national emphysema treatment trial. Chest 2005;128(6):3799–809.

80. Cires-Drouet RS, Mayorga-Carlin M, Toursavadkohi S, et al. Safety of exercise therapy after acute pulmonary embolism. Phlebology 2020;35(10):824–32.

81. Dalal HM, Taylor RS, Jolly K, et al. The effects and costs of home-based rehabilitation for heart failure with reduced ejection fraction: the reach-hf multicentre randomized controlled trial. Eur J Prev Cardiol 2019;26(3):262–72.

82. Hillegass E, Puthoff M, Frese EM, et al. Role of physical therapists in the management of individuals at risk for or diagnosed with venous thromboembolism: Evidence-based clinical practice guideline. Phys Ther 2016;96(2):143–66.

83. Thompson PD. Exercise prescription and proscription for patients with coronary artery disease. Circulation 2005;112(15):2354–63.

84. Wenger NK. Current status of cardiac rehabilitation. J Am Coll Cardiol 2008;51(17):1619–31.

85. Cardiac rehabilitation programs. A statement for healthcare professionals from the American Heart Association. Circulation 1994;90(3):1602–10.

86. Saltin B, Blomqvist G, Mitchell JH, et al. Response to exercise after bed rest and after training. Circulation 1968;38(5 Suppl):VII1–78. Available at: https://www.ncbi.nlm.nih.gov/pubmed/5696236.

87. Naughton J, Lategola MT, Shanbour K. A physical rehabilitation program for cardiac patients: a progress report. Am J Med Sci 1966;252(5):545–53. Available at: https://www.ncbi.nlm.nih.gov/pubmed/5924755.

88. Bethell HJ. Cardiac rehabilitation: from Hellerstein to the millennium. Int J Clin Pract 2000;54(2):92–7.

Available at: https://www.ncbi.nlm.nih.gov/pubmed/10824363.

89. Anderson L, Oldridge N, Thompson DR, et al. Exercise-Based Cardiac Rehabilitation for Coronary Heart Disease: Cochrane Systematic Review and Meta-Analysis. J Am Coll Cardiol 2016;67(1):1–12.

90. Mezzani A, Hamm LF, Jones AM, et al. Aerobic exercise intensity assessment and prescription in cardiac rehabilitation: a joint position statement of the European Association for Cardiovascular Prevention and Rehabilitation, the American Association of Cardiovascular and Pulmonary Rehabilitat. Eur J Prev Cardiol 2013;20(3):442–67.

91. Wisloff U, Stoylen A, Loennechen JP, et al. Superior cardiovascular effect of aerobic interval training versus moderate continuous training in heart failure patients: a randomized study. Circulation 2007;115(24):3086–94.

92. Moholdt T, Aamot IL, Granoien I, et al. Aerobic interval training increases peak oxygen uptake more than usual care exercise training in myocardial infarction patients: a randomized controlled study. Clin Rehabil 2012;26(1):33–44.

93. Taylor JL, Holland DJ, Keating SE, et al. Short-term and Long-term Feasibility, Safety, and Efficacy of High-Intensity Interval Training in Cardiac Rehabilitation: The FITR Heart Study Randomized Clinical Trial. JAMA Cardiol 2020;5(12):1382–9.

94. Guazzi M, Reina G, Tumminello G, et al. Improvement of alveolar-capillary membrane diffusing capacity with exercise training in chronic heart failure. J Appl Physiol 2004;97(5):1866–73.

95. Andrade DC, Arce-Alvarez A, Parada F, et al. Acute effects of high-intensity interval training session and endurance exercise on pulmonary function and cardiorespiratory coupling. Physiol Rep 2020;8(15):e14455.

96. Tasoulis A, Papazachou O, Dimopoulos S, et al. Effects of interval exercise training on respiratory drive in patients with chronic heart failure. Respir Med 2010;104(10):1557–65.

97. Thijssen DH, Dawson EA, Black MA, et al. Brachial artery blood flow responses to different modalities of lower limb exercise. Med Sci Sport Exerc 2009;41(5):1072–9.

98. Calverley TA, Ogoh S, Marley CJ, et al. HIITing the brain with exercise: mechanisms, consequences and practical recommendations. J Physiol 2020;598(13):2513–30.

99. Barnes JN, Schmidt JE, Nicholson WT, et al. Cyclooxygenase inhibition abolishes age-related differences in cerebral vasodilator responses to hypercapnia. J Appl Physiol 2012;112(11):1884–90.

100. Green DJ, Hopman MT, Padilla J, et al. Vascular Adaptation to Exercise in Humans: Role of Hemodynamic Stimuli. Physiol Rev 2017;97(2):495–528.

101. Del Buono MG, Arena R, Borlaug BA, et al. Exercise Intolerance in Patients With Heart Failure: JACC State-of-the-Art Review. J Am Coll Cardiol 2019;73(17):2209–25.

102. Lundby C, Montero D, Joyner M. Biology of VO2 max: looking under the physiology lamp. Acta Physiol 2017;220(2):218–28.

103. Haykowsky MJ, Brubaker PH, Stewart KP, et al. Effect of endurance training on the determinants of peak exercise oxygen consumption in elderly patients with stable compensated heart failure and preserved ejection fraction. J Am Coll Cardiol 2012;60(2):120–8.

104. Levinger I, Bronks R, Cody DV, et al. The effect of resistance training on left ventricular function and structure of patients with chronic heart failure. Int J Cardiol 2005;105(2):159–63.

105. Palevo G, Keteyian SJ, Kang M, et al. Resistance exercise training improves heart function and physical fitness in stable patients with heart failure. J Cardiopulm Rehabil Prev 2009;29(5):294–8.

106. Ozaki H, Loenneke J, Thiebaud R, et al. Resistance training induced increase in VO2max in young and older subjects. Eur Rev Aging Phys Act 2013;10. https://doi.org/10.1007/s11556-013-0120-1.

107. Liu T, Chan AW, Liu YH, et al. Effects of Tai Chi-based cardiac rehabilitation on aerobic endurance, psychosocial well-being, and cardiovascular risk reduction among patients with coronary heart disease: A systematic review and meta-analysis. Eur J Cardiovasc Nurs 2018;17(4):368–83.

108. Borg GA V. Physical Performance and Perceived Exertion. Lund; Copenhagen: Berlingska boktryckeriet, C.W.K. Gleerup ; E. Munksgaard; 1962.

109. Konstantinides SV, Meyer G, Bueno H, et al. 2019 ESC Guidelines for the diagnosis and management of acute pulmonary embolism developed in collaboration with the European respiratory society (ERS). Eur Heart J 2020;41(4):543–603.

110. Ramirez-Jimenez M, Fernandez-Elias V, Morales-Palomo F, et al. Intense aerobic exercise lowers blood pressure in individuals with metabolic syndrome taking antihypertensive medicine. Blood Press Monit 2018;23(5):230–6.

111. Ramirez-Jimenez M, Morales-Palomo F, Ortega JF, et al. Effects of intense aerobic exercise and/or antihypertensive medication in individuals with metabolic syndrome. Scand J Med Sci Sport 2018;28(9):2042–51.

112. Maddison R, Rawstorn JC, Rolleston A, et al. The remote exercise monitoring trial for exercise-based cardiac rehabilitation (REMOTE-CR): A randomised controlled trial protocol. BMC Publ Health 2014;14(1):1–8.

113. Anderson L, Sharp GA, Norton RJ, et al. Home-based versus centre-based cardiac rehabilitation. Cochrane Database Syst Rev 2017;6:CD007130.

114. Bayoumy K, Gaber M, Elshafeey A, et al. Smart wearable devices in cardiovascular care: where we are and how to move forward. Nat Rev Cardiol 2021;18(8):581–99.

Exercise Training in Patients with Chronic Thromboembolic Pulmonary Hypertension and Pulmonary Arterial Hypertension

A Systematic Review and Meta-Analysis of Randomized Controlled Trials

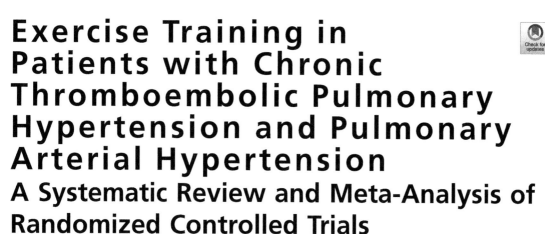

Check for updates

Gabriella VanAken, MD[a,b,*], Drew Rubick, BS[c], Daniel Wieczorek, BS[a],
Saurav Chatterjee, MD[d], Victor M. Moles, MD[e], Prachi P. Agarwal, MD, MS[f],
Jonathan W. Haft, MD[g], Thomas M. Cascino, MD, MSc[e],
Scott H. Visovatti, MD[h], Vikas Aggarwal, MD, MPH[i]

KEYWORDS

• CTEPH • Pulmonary hypertension • Exercise training

KEY POINTS

- In a meta-analysis/systematic review of 5 randomized controlled trials (RCTs) assessing exercise therapy in pulmonary hypertension patients, 20% of whom were diagnosed with chronic thromboembolic pulmonary hypertension (CTEPH), there was a significant improvement in 6-minute walk distance (6MWD) following 3 to 15 weeks of exercise training.
- Exercise training is safe and efficacious, as indicated by the lack of adverse events and improvements in exercise capacity and hemodynamic parameters.
- A limited amount of data assessing exercise training in CTEPH patients is available, including no RCTs investigating exercise training in CTEPH patients exclusively.

[a] University of Michigan Medical School, 1301 Catherine Street, Ann Arbor, MI 48109, USA; [b] Department of Internal Medicine, University of Michigan, 1500 East Medical Center Drive TC 311Q, Ann Arbor, MI 48109, USA; [c] Central Michigan University College of Medical School, 1200 South Franklin Street, Mount Pleasant, MI 48859, USA; [d] Division of Cardiovascular Medicine, North Shore-Long Island Jewish Medical Centers, Northwell Health, Donald and Barbara Zucker School of Medicine at Hofstra/Northwell, 500 Hofstra Boulevard, Hempstead, NY 11549, USA; [e] Division of Cardiology (Frankel Cardiovascular Center), Department of Internal Medicine, University of Michigan, 1425 E Ann Street, Floor 3 Reception C, Ann Arbor, MI 48109, USA; [f] Division of Cardiothoracic Radiology, Department of Radiology, University of Michigan, 1500 East Medical Center Drive, Room 5383, Ann Arbor, MI 48109, USA; [g] Department of Cardiac Surgery, University of Michigan, 1425 East Ann Street, Floor 3 Reception C, Ann Arbor, MI 48109, USA; [h] Department of Cardiovascular Disease, The Ohio State University, 452 West 10th Avenue, 1st Floor, Columbus, OH 43210, USA; [i] Division of Cardiovascular Medicine, Department of Internal Medicine, Henry Ford Hospital, 2799 West Grand Boulevard, K14, Detroit, MI 48202, USA
* Corresponding author. 1500 East Medical Center Drive TC 311Q Ann Arbor, MI 48109.
E-mail address: vanakeng@med.umich.edu

Heart Failure Clin 21 (2025) 137–148
https://doi.org/10.1016/j.hfc.2024.05.003
1551-7136/25/© 2024 Elsevier Inc. All rights are reserved, including those for text and data mining, AI training, and similar technologies.

heartfailure.theclinics.com

INTRODUCTION

Chronic thromboembolic pulmonary hypertension (CTEPH), a subcategory of group 4 pulmonary hypertension (PH), typically presents as exercise intolerance due to persistent skeletal muscle deconditioning, persistent ventilation/perfusion (V/Q) mismatch, ventilatory inefficiency, and PH.[1] The persistent V/Q mismatch leads to inadequate oxygen delivery to activated muscles, causing early onset of fatigue and dyspnea during exercise. Skeletal muscle deconditioning due to chronic inactivity exacerbates these symptoms and causes further impairment in exercise capacity.[1–3]

While it was previously recommended that PH patients, including CTEPH patients, abstain from strenuous physical activity due to concern for worsening clinical outcomes,[4] the use of exercise interventions as a therapeutic option for patients with CTEPH is gaining increased attention.[5] Recent studies have suggested exercise interventions may improve clinical outcomes by improving endothelial function and vascular remodeling, leading to a reduction in pulmonary vascular resistance and improvement in exercise capacity.[6,7] Furthermore, exercise interventions have been shown to decrease systemic inflammation, oxidative stress, and sympathetic nervous system activity, all of which have been associated with the pathophysiology of CTEPH.[8] For these reasons, investigating the efficacy of exercise interventions in improving outcomes in patients with CTEPH is of key clinical interest and could have significant implications for managing this disease.

Previous randomized controlled trials (RCTs) for PH patients have indicated exercise training improves disease-oriented outcomes and patient quality of life (QoL).[5,9] These results have also been extended to CTEPH patients in observational reports. Given the lack of high-quality evidence, it is not surprising that exercise training continues to be underutilized in patients with CTEPH.[2,3,10] By exclusively analyzing RCTs, this study aims to address this knowledge gap and inform the current status of randomized data investigating the efficacy of exercise interventions in patients with CTEPH.

METHODS
Search Strategy and Selection Criteria

A search was conducted using PubMed, EMBASE, and Cochrane for human subject RCTs published prior to January 31, 2023. Keywords used included "exercise," "training," "intervention," "rehabilitation," "pulmonary embolism," "acute PE," "chronic PE," "venous thromboembolic," and "venous thrombo embolic" and "venous thrombo-embolic," "VTE," "chronic thromboembolic" and "chronic thrombo embolic" and "chronic thrombo-embolic," "CTEPH," "thromboembolic disease" and "thrombo embolic disease" and "thrombo-embolic disease," "thromboembolic pulmonary hypertension" and "thrombo embolic pulmonary hypertension" and "thrombo-embolic pulmonary hypertension," "CTED," "chronic pulmonary hypertension," "chronic PH". Inclusion criteria for this meta-analysis were: (1) RCTs with a study population consisting of at least 10% subjects with CTEPH; (2) a study intervention consisting of home or center-based exercise training or rehabilitation lasting at least 3 weeks; (3) change in 6-min walk distance (6MWD) was reported as an outcome; (4) manuscript publication in a peer-reviewed journal (abstracts that were not followed by a full manuscript publication were excluded); (5) study quality, as assessed by Physiotherapy Evidence Database (PEDro) scale, was excellent or good.

Titles, followed by abstracts and full studies, were independently reviewed by 2 authors (G.V. and D.R.) and selected based on inclusion and exclusion criteria. At each stage, a third author (V.A.) resolved discrepancies between the 2 independent reviewer authors (**Fig. 1**).

Outcomes

The primary outcome was the change in 6MWD with exercise intervention. Secondary outcomes included change in peak V_{O_2}, peak workload, health related quality of life (HRQOL), systolic pulmonary artery pressure (sPAP), and the World Health Organization functional classification (WHO-FC).

Data Extraction

Information on study design, quality, location, intervention type, supervision type, duration, outcomes assessed, and characteristics of participants was extracted by 2 authors (G.V. and D.R.) and then independently reviewed by each author for accuracy. Discrepancies were resolved by consensus.

Quality Assessment

Study quality was assessed using the PEDro scale.[11] For this scale, studies with scores of less than 4 are considered "poor," 4 to 5 are considered "fair," 6 to 8 are considered "good," and 9 to 10 are considered "excellent."[12,13]

Statistical Analysis

Excel 2023 and Comprehensive Meta Analysis (CMA) software were used for statistical analyses.

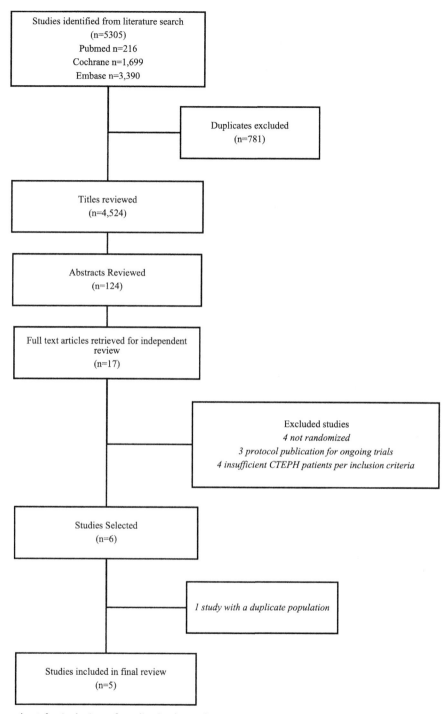

Fig. 1. Flow chart for inclusion of studies in the review.

Using CMA, a Mantel Haenszel fixed and random effects models were used to analyze data quantitatively. Random effects are reported in this analysis. Heterogeneity was assessed using I^2. Continuous data points were analyzed using weighted means, weighted mean differences, and 95% confidence intervals. For studies that only reported pre and post-means and standard deviations, change means were calculated by subtracting the pre from the post-mean, and change standard deviation was calculated assuming a correlation coefficient of 0.5 between pre and post-values as suggested by Buys and colleagues[14]

RESULTS
Study Characteristics

The meta-analysis consisted of 5 RCTs with 293 participants, 58 (20%) diagnosed with CTEPH.[9,15–18] All participants with CTEPH, except those from the trial by Ley and colleagues, had either inoperable or persistent CTEPH after endarterectomy. Ley and colleagues did not specify the operative status of participants in the manuscript. None of the included studies indicated that participants had undergone balloon pulmonary angioplasty (BPA). All studies had participants engage in a supervised exercise program lasting between 3 and 15 weeks. The exercise training was either completed in-hospital or started in-hospital and continued at home. In all 5 included studies, exercise intervention involved aerobic cycle ergometer training, resistance or dumbbell training, and respiratory training. **Table 1** enlists key study characteristics for all studies, including a detailed description of the exercise intervention for each study and medical therapy used.

Quality Assessment

The PEDro scale was used to assess the methodological quality of the included studies (**Table 2**). The researcher responsible for collecting efficacy parameters was blinded to the clinical data in all studies except Ley and colleagues. No significant differences in reported demographic and important clinical characteristics were noted on baseline comparison. A summative assessment of studies revealed 2/5 to be excellent quality and 3/5 to be good quality.

6-Minute Walk Distance

All studies reported the 6MWD for participants at baseline and after exercise intervention.[9,15,16,18] The baseline weighted mean was 445.81 ± 106.15 m for the control participants and 455.51 ± 99.29 m for intervention participants. The post-intervention weighted mean difference was -4.48 ± 51.19 m for control groups and $+41.11 \pm 59.23$ m for intervention participants. Meta-regression demonstrated exercise interventions significantly improved 6MWD with a pooled difference in means of 53.97 ± 13.23 m (P<.01) (**Fig. 2**A). Substantial heterogeneity was also observed on pooled analysis ($I^2 = 71\%$; P<.01). The study by Mereles and colleagues accounted for this noted heterogeneity, and upon exclusion of this study, our results remained largely unchanged (**Fig. 2**B).

Cardiopulmonary Exercise Testing

Peak oxygen consumption

All studies except Ley and colleagues reported CPET results with a baseline weighted mean peak oxygen uptake (Vo_2) of 14.74 ± 4.49 mL/min/kg and 14.05 ± 4.29 mL/min/kg for the control and intervention groups, respectively.[9,16–18] The post-intervention weighted mean difference was -0.18 ± 3.39 mL/min/kg for the control groups and 1.97 ± 2.80 mL/min/kg for the intervention groups. Meta-regression showed a significant improvement in peak Vo_2 with exercise intervention, with a pooled difference in means of 2.33 ± 0.80 mL/min/kg (P<.01) (**Fig. 3**A). Substantial heterogeneity was observed on pooled analysis ($I^2 = 74\%$; P<.01). The study by Grünig and colleagues accounted for this noted heterogeneity, and upon exclusion of this study, our results remained largely unchanged (**Fig. 3**B).

Workload

All studies except Ley and colleagues and González-Saiz and colleagues reported peak workload with baseline weighted means for the control and intervention groups as 70.22 ± 25.56 and 72.51 ± 25.48 W, respectively.[9,16,17] The change in peak workload was 1.27 ± 14.37 W for control groups and 12.47 ± 21.60 W for intervention groups. Meta-regression indicated a trend toward improvement in peak workload with exercise training, with a pooled difference in means of 12.36 ± 6.89 W (P = .07) (**Fig. 4**A). Substantial heterogeneity was observed on pooled analysis ($I^2 = 85\%$; P<.01). The study by Grünig and colleagues accounted for this noted heterogeneity, and upon exclusion of this study, our results remained largely unchanged (**Fig. 4**B).

Pulmonary Artery Systolic Pressure

Grunig and colleagues and Mereles and colleagues used echocardiography to characterize the hemodynamic characteristics of participants before and after exercise training. Pooled analysis demonstrated a sPAP baseline of 61.72 ± 22.67 mm Hg and 64.30 ± 25.49 mm Hg for control and intervention groups with a mean weighted difference of 4.68 ± 17.28 mm Hg and -4.85 ± 14.22 mm Hg respectively. The meta-regression indicated a trend toward reduction in sPAP with exercise training with a pooled difference in means of -4.02 ± 7.22 mm Hg (P = .58) (**Fig. 5**). Significant heterogeneity was observed ($I^2 = 69\%$; P = .07).

Table 1
Study characteristics

Author, Year	Study Population	Baseline WHO-FC	Pulmonary Hypertension Group	Medication Combination Treatment	Exercise Intervention	Duration
Grünig et al, 2021	*Intervention Arm:* n = 58 40/58 (69%) Women Age: 52.3 ±12.4 *Control Arm:* n = 58 45/58 (78%) Women Age: 55 ± 12.7	I: 1 II: 26 III: 30 IV: 1 I: 0 II: 34 III: 24 IV: 0	1: 50/58 (86%) 3: 1/58 (2%) 4: 7/58 (12%) 1: 47/58 (81%) 4: 11/58 (19%)	Monotherapy: 12 (21%) Dual therapy: 24 (41%) Triple therapy: 21 (36%) Quadruple therapy: 1 (2%) Monotherapy: 14 (24%) Dual therapy: 29 (50%) Triple therapy: 15 (26%) Quadruple therapy: 0 (0%)	• Inpatient phase with exercise training 5-7 d/wk consisting of respiratory therapy, cycle ergometer, dumbbell training, and guided walks. • Outpatient phase with exercise training 3-7 d/wk at 40%–60% of maximal workload.	Inpatient: 10–30 d Outpatient: Remaining 15 wk
González-Saiz et al,[18] 2017	*Intervention Arm:* n = 20 12/20 (60%) Women Age: 46 ±11 *Control Arm:* n = 20 12/20 (60%) Women Age: 45 ± 12	N/A N/A	1: 18/20 (90%) 4: 2/20 (10%) 1: 18/20 (90%) 4: 2/20 (10%)	Oral monotherapy: 7 (35%) Combined oral therapy: 7 (35%) Combined oral therapy + prostanoids: 4 (20%) Monotherapy + prostanoids: 2 (10%) Oral monotherapy: 9 (45%) Combined oral therapy: 8 (40%) Combined oral therapy + prostanoids: 3 (15%) Monotherapy + prostanoids: 0 (0%)	• In-hospital cycle ergometer sessions 5 d/wk followed by resistance training sessions 3 d/wk • Inspiratory muscle training 2 times daily, 6 d/wk (morning session in-hospital, evening session at-home)	8 wk
Mereles et al,[16] 2006	*Intervention Arm:* n = 15 5/15 (67%) Women Age: 47 ±12 *Control Arm:* n = 15 5/15 (67%) Women Age: 53 ± 14	II: 4 III: 10 IV: 1 II: 2 III: 12 IV: 1	1: 13/15 (87%) 4: 2/15 (13%) 1: 11/15 (73%) 4: 4/15 (27%)	Monotherapy: 6 (40%) Dual therapy: 5 (33%) Triple therapy: 4 (27%) Monotherapy: 7 (47%) Dual therapy: 5 (33%) Triple therapy: 3 (20%)	• In-hospital training with bicycle ergometer training 7 d/wk at low workloads • 60 min of walking, 30 min of resistance training, and 30 min of respiratory training 5 d/wk	Inpatient: 3 wk Outpatient: 12 wk

(continued on next page)

Table 1
(continued)

Author, Year	Study Population	Baseline WHO-FC	Pulmonary Hypertension Group	Medication Combination Treatment	Exercise Intervention	Duration
					• At-home training with 15–30 min cycle training 5 d/wk, 15–30 min dumbbell and respiratory training every other day, and walking twice per week.	
Ehlken et al, 2016	*Intervention Arm:* n = 46 26/46 (57%) Women Age: 55 ±15	II: 8 III: 36 IV: 0	1: 35/46 (76%) 4: 11/46 (24%)	Monotherapy: 13 (33%) Dual therapy: 20 (51%) Triple therapy: 6 (15%)	• In-hospital training with 1.5 h/day cycle ergometer at low workloads 7 d/wk	Inpatient: 3 wk Outpatient: 12 wk
	Control Arm: n = 41 21/41 (51%) Women Age: 57 ± 15	II: 6 III: 30 IV: 4	1: 26/41 (63%) 4: 15/41 (37%)	Monotherapy: 14 (35%) Dual therapy: 22 (55%) Triple therapy: 4 (10%)	• Walking, dumbbell training, and respiratory training 5 d/wk • Above training continued at home for at least 15 min/day, 5 d/wk	
Ley et al,[15] 2013	*Intervention Arm:* n = 10 8/10 (80%) Women Age: 47 ±8	II: 3 III: 7	1: 9/10 (90%) 4: 1/10 (10%)	Monotherapy: 2 (20%) Dual therapy: 6 (60%) Triple therapy: 2 (20%)	• Same as Mereles	Inpatient: 3 wk
	Control Arm: n = 10 6/10 (60%) Women Age: 54 ± 14	II: 1 III: 9	1: 7/10 (70%) 4: 3/10 (30%)	Monotherapy: 3 (30%) Dual therapy: 6 (60%) Triple therapy: 1 (10%)		

Group 1 = pulmonary arterial hypertension; Group 2 = due to left heart disease; Group 3 = due to lung disease; Group 4 = CTEPH; Group 5 = unclear/multifactorial etiologies.

Table 2
Physiotherapy Evidence Database (PEDro) quality assessment

	Grünig et al,[9] 2021	González-Saiz et al,[18] 2017	Mereles et al,[16] 2006	Ehlken et al,[17] 2016	Ley et al,[15] 2013
Eligibility criteria	Yes	Yes	Yes	No	Yes
Random allocation	Yes	Yes	Yes	Yes	Yes
Concealed allocation	Yes	Yes	Yes	Yes	Yes
Baseline comparability	Yes	Yes	Yes	Yes	Yes
Blinding of participants	No	No	No	No	No
Blinding of therapists	No	No	No	No	No
Blinding of assessors	Yes	Yes	Yes	Yes	No
Adequate follow-up (>85%)	Yes	Yes	Yes	No	Yes
Intention-to-treat analysis	No	Yes	Yes	No	Yes
Between-group statistical comparisons	Yes	Yes	Yes	Yes	Yes
Reporting of point measures and measures of variability	Yes	Yes	Yes	Yes	Yes
	8/11	9/11	9/11	6/11	8/11

Health Related Quality of Life

Two studies, Grunig and colleagues and González-Saiz and colleagues, reported HRQOL physical and mental summation scores obtained using the Short Form 36-Item Health Survey (SF-36).[2,5] Mereles and colleagues reported a significant improvement in mental and physical summation scores. However, this study was not included in the pooled analysis as it did not report pre and post-intervention values.

Physical summation scores

The baseline weighted means were 44.81 ± 17.55 for the control groups and 43.09 ± 16.77 for the intervention groups. No heterogeneity was observed ($I^2 = 0\%$; $P = .95$). The physical summation post-intervention weighted mean differences were 3.48 ± 12.11 for the control groups and 5.74 ± 12.99 for the intervention groups. This difference in physical summation scores with exercise training did not reach statistical significance on meta-regression, with a pooled

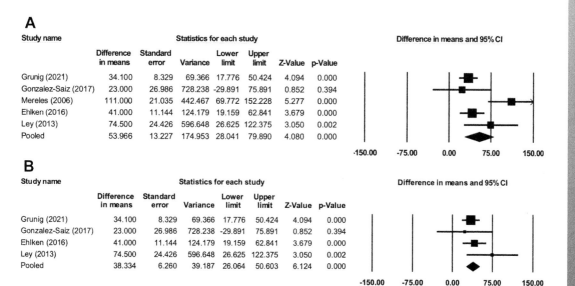

Fig. 2. (*A*) Forest plot showing the effect of exercise intervention on change in 6MWD. (*B*) Forest plot showing the effect of an exercise intervention on change in 6MWD with the exclusion of Mereles and colleagues

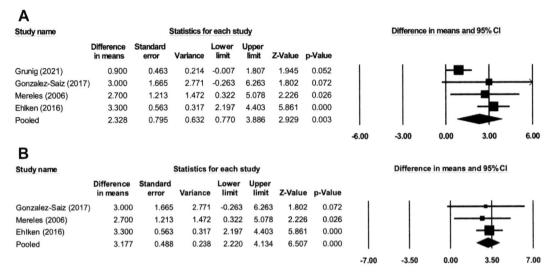

Fig. 3. (*A*) Forest plot showing the effect of exercise intervention on peak Vo$_2$. (*B*) Forest plot showing the effect of an exercise intervention on peak Vo$_2$ with the exclusion of Grünig and colleagues

difference in means of 2.24±1.90 (P = .24) (**Fig. 6**).

Mental summation scores

The baseline weighted means were 55.68±17.34 for the control groups and 55.55±18.90 for the intervention groups, with post-intervention weighted mean differences of 1.95±11.16 for the control groups and 3.94±11.26 for the intervention groups. No heterogeneity was observed (I^2 = 0%; P = .98). This difference in mental summation scores with exercise training did not reach statistical significance on

meta-regression with a pooled difference in means of 2.07±1.94 (P = .29) (**Fig. 7**).

Subscale improvements were seen for select categories in various studies. Ehlken and colleagues demonstrated a significant improvement in vitality score (P = .04); Grünig and colleagues showed a significantly improved mental health score (P<.01), in addition to a trend toward improvement in social function (P = .09) and physical function (P = .07); and Mereles and colleagues reported significant improvements in physical functioning (P = .02), social functioning (P<.01),

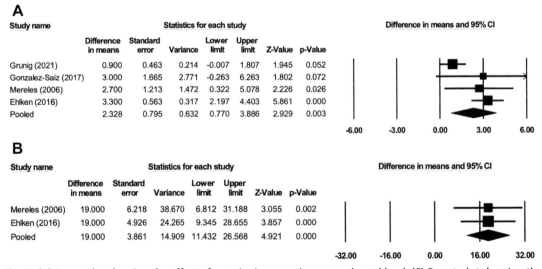

Fig. 4. (*A*) Forest plot showing the effect of exercise intervention on peak workload. (*B*) Forest plot showing the effect of exercise intervention on peak workload with the removal of Grünig and colleagues

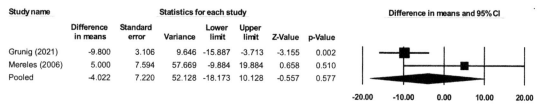

Fig. 5. Forest plot showing the effect of an exercise intervention on sPAP.

role-physical (P<.01), mental health (P<.01), and vitality (P<.01).

World Health Organization Functional Classification

Grünig and colleagues demonstrated significant improvement in WHO-FC, with 9 participants improved and 4 worsened in the training group compared to 1 improved participant and 3 worsened in the control group (P = .03). Mereles' study also reported a significant improvement in WHO-FC at 15 weeks from 2.8±0.6 to 2.3±0.4 in the intervention group, with worsened WHO-FC in the control group from 2.9±0.5 to 3.0±0.3 (P<.01).

Adverse Events

Exercise training overall was well tolerated in the included studies. The pooled dropout rate for exercise intervention participants was 12.75% (19/149). Exercise training was very safe, with no study noting any adverse events attributed to the exercise intervention. 4/149 patients (2.68%) in the intervention arms were noted to experience an arrhythmia during the study interventions; however, none of these events were adjudicated to be exercise-related (**Table 3**). Of note, serious safety events such as worsening right heart failure, syncope, or death due to the exercise interventions were not reported for any patient.

DISCUSSION

The role of exercise training in the management of patients with CTEPH remains understudied, resulting in minimal evidence-based management guidelines for this specific group of PH. As such, this analysis aims to summarize the limited evidence

available to provide an improved understanding of the role of exercise training in the management of patients with CTEPH. Notably, we did not find any RCTs that evaluated the role of exercise training exclusively in patients with CTEPH. Of the 5 RCTs included in this meta-analysis, CTEPH patients constituted 20% (58/293) of the overall PH patient population. Despite small sample sizes, exercise training was remarkably effective and safe in this patient population. Interestingly, the study participants were remarkably compliant with the exercise intervention, as the overall dropout rate was only 12.75% (19/149) in the intervention arm. Notably, the participants with CTEPH were largely considered inoperable at the time of study completion. With the increasing prevalence of BPA as a treatment for CTEPH, many of these participants would have an alternative treatment option aside from medical management.

The results of this study indicate that exercise training is effective at improving exercise capacity, as measured by 6MWD, in patients with PH, including CTEPH. All studies included, except González-Saiz and colleagues, independently demonstrated a significant improvement in 6MWD, with pooled analysis similarly demonstrating a significant improvement in 6MWD in the exercise intervention groups compared to the control groups. Notably, the change in 6MWD observed on pooled analysis (41.11 m) is similar to the reported change in 6MWD with medical management for CTEPH patients.[19] These initial findings suggest that exercise interventions effectively improve exercise capacity and other parameters, as discussed below.

This pooled analysis demonstrated a significant improvement in peak V_{O_2} with exercise intervention and a trend toward improvement in peak workload and sPAP. These results indicate that

Study name	Difference in means	Standard error	Variance	Lower limit	Upper limit	Z-Value	p-Value	Difference in means and 95% CI
Grunig (2021)	2.500	2.763	7.632	-2.915	7.915	0.905	0.365	
Gonzalez-Saiz (2017)	2.000	2.617	6.849	-3.129	7.129	0.764	0.445	
Pooled	2.236	1.900	3.610	-1.487	5.960	1.177	0.239	

Fig. 6. Forest plot showing effect of exercise intervention SF-36 Physical Summation Score.

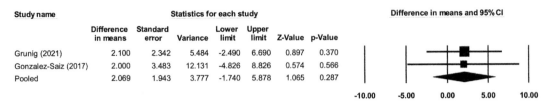

Study name		Statistics for each study						Difference in means and 95% CI
	Difference in means	Standard error	Variance	Lower limit	Upper limit	Z-Value	p-Value	
Grunig (2021)	2.100	2.342	5.484	-2.490	6.690	0.897	0.370	
Gonzalez-Saiz (2017)	2.000	3.483	12.131	-4.826	8.826	0.574	0.566	
Pooled	2.069	1.943	3.777	-1.740	5.878	1.065	0.287	

Fig. 7. Forest plot showing the effect of exercise intervention SF-36 Mental Summation Score.

exercise interventions for CTEPH patients have the potential to improve the disease state of CTEPH participants hemodynamically. These hemodynamic improvements, in addition to the above-noted exercise capacity improvements, are reflected in the significant improvement in WHO-FC noted by Grünig and colleagues and Mereles and colleagues, the studies that included these parameters. However, the lack of blinding is a notable limitation. Similarly, although mental and physical summation, assessed using the SF-36, trended toward improvement with an exercise intervention; these results were not statistically significant on pooled analysis. Additional RCTs for CTEPH patients specifically are needed to further elucidate the effects of exercise interventions for CTEPH patients.

One of the most clinically relevant findings from this analysis is the lack of adverse events caused by the exercise interventions, suggesting that contrary to widespread perception, exercise training is safe in CTEPH and pulmonary arterial hypertension (PAH) patients. It should be noted, however, that all exercise interventions were initiated in the inpatient setting; therefore, the lack of adverse events may be influenced by the controlled setting in which exercise training was started. Therefore, these findings are not necessarily generalizable to all exercise training, particularly exercise training that is exclusively completed at home without the intensive monitoring that inpatient rehabilitation offers. Considering these limitations, the available data

indicates that exercise training is safe in CTEPH patients. This, in addition to the above improvements in exercise capacity, hemodynamic parameters, and HRQOL, suggests that exercise training may be beneficial for CTEPH patients.

These results are in line with the current guideline recommendations to engage PAH and CTEPH patients in supervised exercise training (ESC/ERS PH guidelines 2022 and World PH symposium 2018).[20,21] Guidelines for other cardiopulmonary conditions, such as coronary artery disease and heart failure, have also previously not recommended exercise training but have since been updated to recommend aerobic exercise for improvement in both disease morbidity and mortality.[22] In recent years, the American College of Cardiology has upgraded the level of recommendation for exercise training in PH patients to class 1, level of evidence A,[23] with a subsequent European Respiratory Society statement acknowledging the ability of exercise training to improve exercise capacity, HRQOL, and potentially right ventricular function.[24] Most recently, the American Thoracic Society Clinical Practice Guideline also supported pulmonary rehabilitation for patients with PH; however, it noted that this intervention should be considered only for stable patients who are optimized on medical therapy.[25] Despite these advances, exercise interventions are not universally recommended for CTEPH patients and are typically not covered by insurance.[24]

Table 3
Adverse events noted in exercise training participants

Study	Total Number of Exercise Training Participants	Exercise-Related Adverse Events	Arrhythmias (None Found to be due to Exercise Intervention)
Grünig	58	None	3
González-Saiz	20	None	1
Mereles	15	None	0
Ehlken	46	Adverse events not mentioned	0[a]
Ley	10	Adverse events not mentioned	0[a]

[a] If adverse events were not reported, we assumed none occurred.

The lack of RCTs aimed at assessing the potential benefits of exercise training in patients with CTEPH is notable; our study emphasizes the need for such studies.

SUMMARY

This study indicates exercise training may be effective and safe in patients with PH, including CTEPH. Notably, there is a need for RCTs investigating the efficacy and safety of exercise training for CTEPH patients, given the lack of studies exclusively investigating exercise training in this population.

CLINICS CARE POINTS

- Exercise training appears to be safe and effective in CTEPH patients, based on the limited data available.
- Further studies investigating exercise training in CTEPH patients are needed.

LIMITATIONS

One of the most notable limitations of this study is that none of the studies included separate results for CTEPH patients versus other groups of PH. Our analysis is unique in its selective inclusion of only RCTs. However, to the authors' knowledge, there are no RCTs for exercise interventions where results are selectively reported for CTEPH patients. Therefore, this study assumes that the outcomes reported are similar to those of the CTEPH participant subgroups. Secondly, 4/5 of the included studies were single-center studies, indicating that larger, multicenter studies are needed for generalizability. Thirdly, the included studies did not have long-term follow-ups, preventing continued assessment of the effects of exercise interventions for these patients. Fourthly, included studies had bias risk from lack of subject or exercise therapist blinding, which was prohibited by the nature of the study. Finally, as with all meta-analyses, bias cannot be excluded.

DISCLOSURE

The authors have nothing to disclose.

REFERENCES

1. Kim NH, Delcroix M, Jais X, et al. Chronic thromboembolic pulmonary hypertension. Eur Respir J 2019; 53(1):1801915.

2. Fukui S, Ogo T, Takaki H, et al. Efficacy of cardiac rehabilitation after balloon pulmonary angioplasty for chronic thromboembolic pulmonary hypertension. Heart 2016;102(17):1403–9.

3. La Rovere MT, Pinna GD, Pin M, et al. Exercise training after pulmonary endarterectomy for patients with chronic thromboembolic pulmonary hypertension. Respiration 2019;97(3):234–41.

4. Galiè N, Torbicki A, Barst R, et al. Guidelines on diagnosis and treatment of pulmonary arterial hypertension. The Task Force on Diagnosis and Treatment of Pulmonary Arterial Hypertension of the European Society of Cardiology. Eur Heart J 2004;25(24): 2243–78.

5. Chan L, Chin LMK, Kennedy M, et al. Benefits of intensive treadmill exercise training on cardiorespiratory function and quality of life in patients with pulmonary hypertension. Chest 2013;143(2):333–43.

6. Fox BD, Kassirer M, Weiss I, et al. Ambulatory rehabilitation improves exercise capacity in patients with pulmonary hypertension. J Card Fail 2011;17(3): 196–200.

7. Grünig E, Lichtblau M, Ehlken N, et al. Safety and efficacy of exercise training in various forms of pulmonary hypertension. Eur Respir J 2012;40(1):84–92.

8. Richter MJ, Grimminger J, Krüger B, et al. Effects of exercise training on pulmonary hemodynamics, functional capacity and inflammation in pulmonary hypertension. Pulm Circ 2017;7(1):20–37.

9. Grünig E, MacKenzie A, Peacock AJ, et al. Standardized exercise training is feasible, safe, and effective in pulmonary arterial and chronic thromboembolic pulmonary hypertension: results from a large European multicentre randomized controlled trial. Eur Heart J 2021;42(23):2284–95.

10. Nagel C, Prange F, Guth S, et al. Exercise training improves exercise capacity and quality of life in patients with inoperable or residual chronic thromboembolic pulmonary hypertension. PLoS One 2012; 7(7):e41603.

11. de Morton NA. The PEDro scale is a valid measure of the methodological quality of clinical trials: a demographic study. Aust J Physiother 2009;55(2): 129–33.

12. Gonzalez GZ, Moseley AM, Maher CG, et al. Methodologic quality and statistical reporting of physical therapy randomized controlled trials relevant to musculoskeletal conditions. Arch Phys Med Rehabil 2018;99(1):129–36.

13. Foley NC, Teasell RW, Bhogal SK, et al. Stroke rehabilitation evidence-based review: Methodology. Top Stroke Rehabil 2003;10(1):1–7.

14. Buys R, Avila A, Cornelissen VA. Exercise training improves physical fitness in patients with pulmonary arterial hypertension: a systematic review and meta-analysis of controlled trials. BMC Pulm Med 2015;15:40.

15. Ley S, Fink C, Risse F, et al. Magnetic resonance imaging to assess the effect of exercise training on pulmonary perfusion and blood flow in patients with pulmonary hypertension. Eur Radiol 2013; 23(2):324–31.

16. Mereles D, Ehlken N, Kreuscher S, et al. Exercise and respiratory training improve exercise capacity and quality of life in patients with severe chronic pulmonary hypertension. Circulation 2006;114(14):1482–9.

17. Ehlken N, Lichtblau M, Klose H, et al. Exercise training improves peak oxygen consumption and haemodynamics in patients with severe pulmonary arterial hypertension and inoperable chronic thrombo-embolic pulmonary hypertension: a prospective, randomized, controlled trial. Eur Heart J 2016;37(1):35–44.

18. González-Saiz L, Fiuza-Luces C, Sanchis-Gomar F, et al. Benefits of skeletal-muscle exercise training in pulmonary arterial hypertension: The WHOLEi+12 trial. Int J Cardiol 2017;231:277–83.

19. Chen Y, Li F, Luo J, et al. Comparative efficacy and safety of targeted therapies for chronic thromboembolic pulmonary hypertension: a systematic review and network meta-analysis. Can Respir J 2021; 2021:1626971.

20. Desai SA, Channick RN. Exercise in patients with pulmonary arterial hypertension. J Cardiopulm Rehabil Prev 2008;28(1):12–6.

21. Humbert M, Kovacs G, Hoeper MM, et al. 2022 ESC/ERS Guidelines for the diagnosis and treatment of pulmonary hypertension. Eur Respir J 2023;61(1): 2200879.

22. Thompson PD, Buchner D, Pina IL, et al. Exercise and physical activity in the prevention and treatment of atherosclerotic cardiovascular disease: a statement from the Council on Clinical Cardiology (Subcommittee on Exercise, Rehabilitation, and Prevention) and the Council on Nutrition, Physical Activity, and Metabolism (Subcommittee on Physical Activity). Circulation 2003;107(24):3109–16.

23. Galiè N, Humbert M, Vachiery JL, et al. 2015 ESC/ERS Guidelines for the diagnosis and treatment of pulmonary hypertension: the joint task force for the diagnosis and treatment of pulmonary hypertension of the european society of cardiology (ESC) and the European Respiratory Society (ERS): endorsed by: Association for European Paediatric and Congenital Cardiology (AEPC), International Society for Heart and Lung Transplantation (ISHLT). Eur Heart J 2016;37(1):67–119.

24. Grünig E, Eichstaedt C, Barberà JA, et al. ERS statement on exercise training and rehabilitation in patients with severe chronic pulmonary hypertension. Eur Respir J 2019;53(2):1800332.

25. Rochester CL, Alison JA, Carlin B, et al. Pulmonary rehabilitation for adults with chronic respiratory disease: an official american thoracic society clinical practice guideline. Am J Respir Crit Care Med 2023;208(4):e7–26.

Printed and bound by CPI Group (UK) Ltd, Croydon, CR0 4YY

08/05/2025

01864747-0012